The Human Aura

Reading Auras & Colors

Davina DeSilver

Copyright © 2013 Davina DeSilver

All rights reserved.

DEDICATION

To my daughters;
You blessed my life with a color that is unique & a glow
that will warm my heart forever

CONTENTS

1	You Can Read Auras	1
2	Reading Auras	5
3	The Human Energy System	9
4	The Red Aura	12
5	The Orange Aura	20
6	The Yellow Aura	26
7	The Green Aura Personality	33
8	The Blue Aura Personality Type	44
9	The Indigo Aura	53
10	The Violet Aura	62
11	The Crystal Aura	72
12	Pink In The Aura	77
13	Brown In The Aura	80
14	Chakras - The Energy Centers of The Aura	83
15	Start Reading Auras	94
16	The Magic Matrix	106
17	Seeing, Scanning & Sensing Auras	111

ACKNOWLEDGMENTS

To the many clients who allowed me to read their energy and bared their soul to me. Also to those that 'encouraged' me to stand up and share what I have seen. Without you this would not have been possible.

Thank you.

The Human Aura - Reading Auras & Colors

1 YOU CAN READ AURAS

To be able to read auras, many people assume you have to be born with a gift. Well in my view we all were, we just forgot how to use it. To read auras, you need to converse with energy, and as with any conversation you need to know the language. You *can* learn the language of energy.

This language is not restricted to words; it includes images and pictures, much like the very first civilizations used images and symbols to communicate meaning. It also includes feeling and sound for some people. Having some kind of alphabet will help, otherwise your ability to communicate is pretty limited but this is less about learning, than it is about allowing.

This is a very subjective and intuitive topic but also you need something to draw upon. This first book is all about giving you some of those basics. It's like a lot of things in life; learn the basics initially, in some cases the rules and then you can kind of let them go. Information seems to flow to you and through you; and for me I often find I'm speaking words I had no prior knowledge I was going to say. What happens for me is I start from the basics that I'll share with you here and suddenly the images and color of spirit take over, it's as if a video starts playing in my mind and I simply relate back as best I can, what I see and feel to the person in front of me.

From what I've seen, many people try to read an aura by expecting to see a pretty colored bubble hovering around someone. Don't expect to see it with your eyes, certainly not immediately. This can be the very thing that blocks you, your own expectation of how it 'should' be.

There is no 'should' here. I'm sharing what works for me, others may have different approaches but I have found this to be incredibly successful and is something I believe we can all do. Rather than 'see' - by staring hard at the person or trying to go cross eyed at them whilst you try to let your eyes go out of focus, let yourself feel it, experience it, just as you can feel and experience a memory, that's the way you'll 'see' it. This is also how you'll know it's not you just imagining it; you will get strong feelings, sensations and sometimes emotions.

I'll cover that more in depth in the future, for now let's get going on this amazing journey and although that term is overused, you know what, it *is* a journey as to really read and understand auras, you have to read and understand people, yourself and the nature of the human spirit as well as the energy that connects all things.

Your interest in auras is a colorful way of you dancing with your spirit and appreciating the beautiful language of energy and the endless pictures it can paint.

So Why Bother to Read Auras?

For some people it's purely about entertainment, for some it's intriguing and interesting. For me it's something more. It's an effective way of introducing someone to the idea, they are more than just a physical body. That their seemingly non-existent energy fields are holding on to so much about them as an individual, and that these fields can be changed and enhanced.

When I relay back to them events or situations I see and feel, that I would have no way of knowing about, they want to find out more. They want to know if they can do it for themselves.

Their energy body and the care of it, becomes a part of their life and interest. This then can lead on to them wanting to find out about the existence of their spirit and soul. I know when I have sat at workshops and started talking to one person about touching my spirit and helping others to do the same, I often look up and find I have several other interested people huddled around me, wanting to know more too.

To me, when we start talking with and about our spirit, our soul, our higher self, call it what you will, we start to see the bigger picture in our lives and the part we play in that picture. In fact not only do we get to see that we *are* the picture, we see we are the artist, the brush and the paint! Well then it's not too far away to suggest that should we see a picture we don't really like that much, we can start to paint it differently.

So, although this book is an introduction to reading auras, with it aimed towards an entertaining interest for many people, it is my hope that for a few it becomes something more, but for all, I trust that it is worthwhile.

2 READING AURAS

To read an aura, we need to appreciate what it is made of, it's past and its potential. We live in a vibratory universe, we were taught that at school, what we see and touch, although it may seem and feel fixed and solid, is made up of billions of tinier atoms and molecules, none of which are static.

Don't worry you don't need to be scientific; this book is anything but scientific. But the human spirit, you as a person, an entity, you don't finish at your skin. One thing that makes us so very human is our emotions, good, bad and indifferent. These feelings and emotions all have an energy to them, you know you have felt things about people, without them having to say a word. You can feel the different energy in a word said in a venomous way and the beautiful energy in a wonderful hymn or uplifting song.

Really it's not about learning how to read, it's about learning how the information is put together. You learn the process and as you get your thinking mind out of the way by keeping it busy with concentrating on what it knows, you open yourself up so you can more clearly interpret what's really going on, using more of your subconscious mind.

But in order to be able to do that we need to have some basic framework to build from and I am hoping I can really start from the basics in this initial book and if it interests you, it can be something you will build on and you'll evolve in your own personal way with it.

To successfully read and understand the aura, you almost need to be able to wear each color as a cloak and with that cloak comes its own particular characteristics and personality traits. Now that's not to say each Red person is exactly the same, just as with any personality traits, that is not so, there is a potential of similarities and areas of interest that may be the same.

What is important is that you know the potential areas, the aspects that usually sit hand in hand with each color and the corresponding chakra. With this bank of knowledge, your mind will have far more to pull from, when you are ready to read the aura. Then what you will find is that you are instinctively drawn to the aspects that are relevant and important for each individual client.

Just as if you were reading similarities between men and women and areas of interest for example, broadly speaking we might say that men are more interested in football and motor sports than women. That doesn't mean that no women are interested in either of those things. When you are working with the aura and any psychic related area, it is important to set aside your own assumptions and judgments, this is about honestly and cleanly accepting information that is there, without adding your own personal slant to it.

That is where things can go wrong, where misguided good intentions can be misleading and you might find people cannot relate to what it is you have to say.

It can be hard, certainly initially to be brave enough to just say what comes into your mind, but give it a go and just trust as much as you can. I know when I started I held back so often, only to find that had I been brave enough to verbalize the images and impressions I was getting, the client could perfectly relate to what I'd seen.

On the converse don't get drawn into the trap of just making anything up and letting your imagination run riot. You'll soon know what is relevant, certain areas will stand out more than others and as you look deeper, short stories unfold that the person in front of you can relate to. In that story will be some learning, some understanding for that person, regardless of whether they want to share that with you or not, so don't look for answers and fixed results. It doesn't need to make sense for you - just them. Be content with a nod of the head, be careful not to probe into situations or events that are none of your concern, unless the client wishes to delve deeper themselves.

You also need to be very sensitive and aware of what you are saying, more so when you are reading at a deeper level, as some very emotional and fragile things can come up, which the client may or may not wish to discuss. Remember this is not a therapy, there is no 'fixing' involved and I would set your intention to keep things light hearted, certainly whilst learning this skill. Although reading auras for me is more than entertainment, for our purposes here, we'll keep it at the fun and entertaining level!

Don't block your progress by expecting to have to see a brightly colored bubble around every person. That's just your own need for proof, let it go. Try not to have fixed expectations, just be open to taking in this knowledge, using it as a guide and then start sharing what you see with your family and friends. Have fun with it!

3 THE HUMAN ENERGY SYSTEM

The Human Energy Body

In energy terms, we speak of different bodies, subtle energy systems; not only do we have the physical body but we have the emotional, the mental and the spiritual body as well.

These fit together very much like the systems within our physical frame, we have the muscular system, the skeletal system, the endocrine system and the respiratory system. They all fit together and merge, to sustain the whole body, well so it is with the energy body.

It is always trying to maintain balance just like the human body; it is a perfect operating system. The energy body is fed by energy centers called chakras, these feed the aura, which is what you'll be reading and interpreting.

We can read it because whenever there's a malfunction or blockage or something is not right, the energy starts telling a story. When we look at that story it can be very revealing and insightful, to me it is just another way that your subconscious mind uses to bring things to your conscious attention and awareness.

We all got so clever and intelligent in our modern world, we thought we'd lost a lot of our intuitive senses, but we haven't lost them - we just haven't listened to them much. If you start listening and paying attention, you'll be amazed at what you can learn.

The human energy system is an intricate work of art. For our purposes here though, we will keep it simple. There are seven main centers in the energy body and it is these that feed and make up the aura. These go right from the base of the spine to the top of the head. These energy centers or chakras all work together, forever opening and closing, taking energy in, and giving it back-out. They are constantly sensing, they also resonate with specific sounds, and colors.

You'll never stop learning about the chakras, so don't allow yourself to get overwhelmed. I've included some basics in the chapter: Chakras - The Energy Centers of the Aura. It is often one of these main seven colors that you will come across when reading auras, which are easy to remember as they are the colors of the rainbow:

Red, Orange, Yellow, Green, Blue, Indigo, Violet

I've also included brown, pink and white as these can confuse people, when they come across them in the aura.

You'll find there is a chapter on each of these colors, describing the personality traits and characteristics you might expect associated with them. These are not cast in stone but as you'll see, they will be your starting point and with each person, some of the attributes will feel relevant and will come to mind, when you are reading for someone and some won't.

We'll go through each of the colors, their attributes and traits, and then we'll delve deeper into the body matrix, so that you have a good base of knowledge to call upon.

We'll also discuss a few ethical considerations and how you can sit in your energetic body in a place of compassion and non judgment so that you can far easily read and interpret someone else's energy and even you own.

4 THE RED AURA

The Personality Traits of the Red Aura:

There are some colors that have more noticeable shades and tones within them, which when attributed to the aura can signify different aspects of character and personality traits associated with them. Red is one of these colors and for our purposes here, I'll record the most common personality traits mainly of the bright red shade and briefly mention the attributes of the Darker Reds. Know that it is not necessary to tick every single box but you'll instinctively feel if these characteristics relate to you (or your client, if you are reading for somebody else).

The Red personality is a doer; they are active, dynamic people with a zest and energy for life. They are motivated and like to see results. They can be very driven and goal orientated. They like to see physical results for their achievements, so can like practical jobs and chores, like mowing the lawn for example, where the result is immediate and quite gratifying for them.

In their profession, they can be attracted to a sales and target driven environment, they will often be team leaders or managers and will enjoy seeing graphs and charts of progress and will be motivated to reach and exceed those targets. They respond well to the visual stimulus and reminders of why they are engaged in a process. They relate well to information displayed in this more tangible way and may not be drawn to more emotive based professions, like therapy or counseling.

Reds are often kinesthetic, in that they like an aspect of physicality about their profession - some form of movement, they may be gym instructors, personal trainers, or in the armed forces even. In business they may be sales people, out on the rounds, meeting customers face to face and creating contacts whilst meeting targets.

Reds like money because it enables them to do the things they want and they have an entrepreneurial air to them, they don't tend to like being told what to do and may push boundaries and established ways of thinking. They can often be found running their own business, or self employed; in charge of their own destiny, enjoying the fruits of their labor.

These people tend to be pretty sociable, often with a full diary or schedule of things to do and get done. They want to live life and enjoy their experiences and understand that they are responsible for creating those. They may have the odd 'duvet day' but by and large they are few and far between as it doesn't suit their character to sit still for too long. They want to know what it is to be alive.

For some, that means they know how to enjoy life and live it how they'd like, they enjoy success and may be very driven, more so than their other family members at home.

They can be quite impetuous and might not be known for their patience. If they have decided that something is right, they want it now or at least they want to start working towards it now. They like to know a process has been started that will bring them closer to their goal. There will always be things, these people would like to do or places they'd like to visit. These are the inventors of the bucket list!

Reds are energetic, lively types that respond well to physical activity, they find it a great way to let off steam and if they are cooped up too much and not able to physically release their tension, then they could build up like a pressure cooker. And they can have frequent outbursts of frustration or temper.

They literally need to let off steam and it is important for them to be very aware of exactly what works for them, to be able to do this effectively and positively. It might be a session in the gym, a long run outdoors or some type of sports activity that physically pushes them as their tension will definitely be felt and stored in the muscles and nerves if not released. Reds can easily build up a sense of frustration if they have been relatively inactive for a while and may not have made that conscious connection that they feel so much better after a period of activity.

The Red Personality, although they tend to be pretty sociable, can be very independent and even judgmental, it is not easy for them to comprehend how others might not be so motivated or focused as them. They will often prefer to do things themselves rather than delegate, as they don't usually feel that others will do quite as good a job as them. "If I want it done properly, I'll do it myself" can be a common motto.

Reds tend to be very aware of their physical body and will take care of it; some may go to extremes and become obsessed by looks and nutrition, aiming for perfection. They are also aware of other people's bodies, so tend to like being around other attractive, active and/or successful people.

The Red Personality likes to socialize with likeminded individuals, which can be an extension of the people they work alongside, such as other team members if they are professional sports people, dancers or others within the same profession. So although they can be individualistic in their thinking they also like the ambience of the group energy which is usually a dynamic group.

Young people will often display a red aura as they have a lot of vibrant energy running through them.

Red Relationships

Sex is usually pretty high on the scale of importance of the Red personality, that's in quality and quantity. A good, enjoyable and active sex life is often one of the ways they define their success. Sex is a great release for Reds and helps to cultivate a sense of satisfaction for them.

The act of sex has great significance and is again one way they have of feeling a physical sense of success and love. They are by no means emotionally deprived, it is merely that the physical act of intimacy is key to their sense of wellbeing as such an active and dynamic personality type, whereas some other colors are content with companionship and need a meeting of minds more than physical lovemaking to feel safe and secure.

These active types do have feelings and are surprisingly sensitive; however they won't usually show just how sensitive they are. They may not be used to verbally expressing their emotions and may even shy away from doing so. Their partners may feel a little excluded or shut out, as they won't often engage in intimate talk and emotional exploration, certainly not as much as they will physically make love.

In fact they can feel quite awkward about such matters, this is not to say they never will, but it is usually not something they are used to and might be one of the areas they will want to work on to enjoy a healthy long term relationship. They tend to favor doing something rather than verbal communication and this is one of their characteristics that their partners and co-workers need to understand.

This can be one of the reasons, some Reds struggle with longer relationships; they love the power and dynamism, the excitement and thrill of the initial attraction. The sexuality and the energy of a new relationship can be quite addictive for them. So they can move from relationship to relationship, which might have suited them for a while but to enjoy a long term positive partnership, they may need to embrace the emotions not just of themselves but of their partners too and become more conversant about how they feel.

Deep Red Aura

With a deeper shade of red in the aura, these people may well be more manual workers, physically working with their hands and their physical labor is their source of income. There is a slightly slower feel to this shade of red, than of the bright vibrant tone. They may not be so bothered about their own personal appearance but they have a strength and stamina about them.

These people are dependable and reliable. They enjoy the satisfaction of hard work and physical toil. They may have larger hands than other colors; they use their sense of touch and the dexterity of their hands is often their source of income and means of survival. They are practical and down to earth.

They may not be so driven in a goal orientated, achievement kind of way but they will stay the course and work to get the job done. They may not be the first to finish but they will produce good work and are solid personality types, a strong foundation for the family unit. Dependable and reliable are words that spring to mind.

Hopefully that has given you a flavor of the Red personality type. It's important to be aware of the chakra characteristics that this color relates to as it will increase your understanding of the Red Aura and it will also allow you to give more accurate and detailed readings. In the chapter on Chakras you'll find information to get you started.

It's important to get a good feel for what each color means, the highs and the lows, how each characteristic might have two extremes, for example:

Having a good level of energy to get things done might be the happy medium, take it down and you have lethargy and a lack of motivation, turn it up and you might be pushing yourself and others too hard, maybe being seen as aggressive and pushy.

Keywords Associated with the Red Aura Color:

- Passion & Vitality
- Survival
- Strength
- Stamina
- Physical Health & Body
- Manifestation
- Success
- Sex
- Vibrant
- Energy
- Grounded
- Sociable yet Individual
- Core Relationships
- Safety
- Power

There are positive and negative potentials with every energy center and with every color and at times we need the energy of anger for example to change a situation. Having a list of attributes or areas to consider when reading the aura, is a starting point. You'll find a link to a downloadable list of attributes on the Resource page at the end of this book.

Combining this later with how to sense the energy, will enable you to then determine the shade or tone of the color to better understand what is going on and what is relevant to the person in front of you. You'll know if the color feels bright and strong or weak and restricted and then be able to convey a more accurate message and reading.

5 THE ORANGE AURA

Although the Orange Personality shows very similar characteristics to vibrant Reds, these people thrive on challenging their minds as well as their physical body. They are stimulated by adventure and the thrill of experiences as well as the creative strategies they employ to achieve their wants and desires. They combine analytical thinking with an exuberant and creative energy that can be exhilarating to be around.

These people have an adventurous spirit, they are not tied to physical action, and they can be creative and inspiring in how they go about their lives. They can get quite involved in the intricacies and planning process of making things happen and accomplishing their next challenge. This is less about a one off challenge, as much as their attitude to life in general. If they are not an obviously active person in physical ways, they are usually mentally active and very intelligent types. Their energy is involved in creating; evolving new concepts and ideas.

They can be very organized and methodical about the steps involved in making their dreams and plans come true. They like to be involved in the creative process of making things a reality and will not want to sit back and let others make all the decisions.

As such, they dislike handing over control to others and can sometimes come across as selfish as they don't tend to involve them in the planning process very much. They like to ensure they get the most enjoyment out of their activities and therefore want to handle the planning to avoid potential disappointment. They don't expect others to know what they want and need so just don't tend to stop and think that the people around them might like to be a bit more involved too.

They love the adrenaline of adventure and risk, and can almost become addicted to it, seeming to continually need another challenge or risky situation to feel alive. For some Orange types, they are less addicted to adrenaline as they could be to other things that can give them a high, such as: food, drugs, alcohol, and gambling, smoking and even relationships.

These people like being stimulated, they will usually like to travel to new places, to taste new cultures and try new things. They are driven by their likes and dislikes and are usually very clear on what they do and don't like.

Again, to the people around them, this can seem selfish but it is not driven by a selfish need, it is more a pleasant curiosity they have about life and the only sure way they have to determine if they do or don't like something is to experience it. They don't want to be told by somebody else that this or that is good, they want to try it for themselves and they want to keep on experiencing good things.

The Orange Personality can be found throughout the business world, they are rarely stuck for an idea or a new way of doing things. They'll try something out and test it live rather than allow a novel idea to be quashed by doubters. This isn't just blind optimism as they have an analytical aspect to their nature and will have given thought to proposals and plans but are also willing to take a risk.

They can be emotionally intelligent and can seem to just 'get' people, they appreciate the many factors involved in human behavior, so can usually manage people pretty well. However they don't always manage to transfer that across in their closest relationships, as that level of intimacy and bonding can seem to slow them down. This can be true even in their own personal relationship with themselves, as it can be a tough journey to embark upon.

One of the challenges that faces the Orange Personality is to not chase and settle for surface pleasures; sometimes the thrill of planning and the excitement of the idea can mean their minds are so active about what is coming next, the next big thrill, that they somehow miss out on tasting the full flavor of what it is they are doing now. So what seemed like it was going to be great fun or a delicious experience in reality, can suddenly seem a little tame or bland, so they start working on the next big thing, exhausting and frustrating their nearest and dearest and those closest to them.

Basically they just want to enjoy life, so can be great fun to know and be around, they just have to be careful that they actually allow themselves to experience the fun and absorb it on a deeper level, as it is all too easy for them to become chasers of a great time rather than actually getting to enjoy what it is they were planning. I suppose the easiest thing I can liken that to, is running yourself a deep warm bath, thinking you might enjoy a good old soak and the reality is after 2 minutes sat in the tub, you get all fidgety, feel bored and decide to get out, wishing you'd just had a shower instead.

They are often drawn to extreme sports or team pursuits and careers that require physical action combined with strategic thinking too. They are less driven by material success as an *internal* measure of success and a satisfaction. That may be physical or a mental satisfaction and recognition that they have conquered some challenge. Careers that present new challenges, requiring new creative thinking fit very well with the Orange character.

The Orange personality can be found in a wide range of careers, from business, to sports, to academic positions requiring analytical thinking or coming up with creative solutions of one form or another. Even scientific or psychology based careers and interests.

Strangely, these people although they like new challenges, they can also have fixed habits and rituals. They may have a certain process they go through, or like specific things just so, as they like daily 'small' matters to remain the same and constant, so that they don't distract from the main work of the day. For example, they may have particular days of the week for chores, or a certain breakfast or dressing regime, that if threatened or questioned, they can be very protective about.

Orange in Relationships

As a personality type they don't tend to need people around quite so much as other aura colors. They are independent and not that bothered by other people's thoughts and judgments. This again can mean they are perceived as being a little self-centered. They don't feel they have to conform to all the rules of society, sometimes it's like they think rules are made with other people in mind.

They tend to be fit and attractive personalities, so they usually have admirers around them and will not have a problem with creating relationships, though they will soon move on if things become too heavy and if they feel hampered or restricted in any way. They also like quite a lot of time to themselves in a relationship, which is not always easy for their partner. They might come across as disinterested in other people.

If out of balance, not in flow with their positive creativity the Orange type can become manipulative and controlling. They can become very jealous as the stifled emotional power gets angry and annoyed if it sees others doing what they feel they can't.

These are creative thinkers and can feel stifled if they are not stimulated or challenged in which case they can almost seem to shut off and shut down. If their creativity is blocked they can become stifled and may struggle to find a solution. The excitement and natural curiosity for life is the life blood for this personality type, one of their challenges can be trying to balance this need of theirs and the needs and wants of the other people around them. They can seem to spend a lot of time, in their own mind, occupied by their own thoughts.

Keywords for the Orange Personality:

- Creativity
- Ideas
- Analytical and Logical Thinking
- Flow
- Desires
- Emotions
- Activity & Strategy
- Habits & Rituals
- Addictions
- Stimulation

6 THE YELLOW AURA

This lovely bright sunshine color denotes the many wonderful attributes of the Yellow Personality. They are like little rays of sunshine; people seem to be naturally attracted to their warm and sunny disposition.

They have a playful attitude to life and often have an innocence about them and can seem younger than their years, often physically ageing very well. That is not to say they are childish, but they retain a childlike quality in things, an interest and wonder about life. They are easily interested and inspired.

Unfortunately this can sometimes make them an easy target for fraudsters as they can believe the best in people and can be easily taken in by a good story. This is especially possible when they are displaying signs of being out of power, as they are a power color and generally have very good gut instincts and reactions.

These people have a bright sense of humor, a keen mind and intellect. They can be addictive multi-taskers, always with ideas and projects on the go. The thing to watch out for and ask these people is not how many projects are on the go but how many do you finish?

Yellows have the spark and the fire to get projects off the ground and as such, make great inspirers and team leaders; however they can lose motivation and energy further into the project. They find that dealing with detail and process a bit on the boring side and may want to skip a couple of steps, eager to start on the next new thing.

There is a spontaneity about them and they are very sensitive to other people and their environment. They are in touch with the physical body and make good healers and counselors. By nature they are very sympathetic and can maintain a bright attitude even in the hardest of circumstances.

Yellows are entertainers, aware of the ambience and feel of a room and atmosphere. They feel happy when the vibes are good and buoyant and they will strive to keep them that way.

They love having fun and want others to experience that too. They love to laugh and will always encourage and entice others to laugh with them. They don't want to take life too seriously and will often be inviting other people to do the same.

They can be very sociable people and are often well liked by others. They will usually have lots of friends and acquaintances but can probably count on one hand the number of people they truly confide in.

This stems from not wanting to be bogged down by the heaviness of life, they don't want to burden others with their problems. The danger is of course, presenting a happy smiling face to the world whilst their deepest concerns go along unaddressed.

These people are very kinesthetic, they respond to touch and can be very tactile. They can really enjoy meditation and spiritual practices as they feel such a sense of pleasure and enjoyment from them. They also learn by doing and trying things, rather than pure instruction. They like to know how something feels to be able to really get to grips with it.

Any physical activities they do will also have an element of fun such as beach volley ball, surfing or swimming. A sense of physical freedom can be important to Yellows. This can follow through into their work life and careers as they make great free-lancers or will enjoy self employment of one kind or another. They are not driven by money, rather they view it as a necessity, so they will earn it but they prefer to work at something they enjoy. They can earn and spend money quite easily but it might go as quick as it comes at times.

They can be very quick witted, and will usually have a comic reply that effortlessly seems to roll out, endearing themselves with workmates and people around them. They will also be very quick in their speech pattern; sometimes it can be hard to follow as the words just seem to keep on coming when they are in flow.

Yellows can ignore problems and challenges, they have various means of doing that, excessive sleeping, lethargy, continually moving from one location to another or just keeping very busy, particularly with all the things that don't really matter. Some Yellows are continually late and will always have a great excuse. They dislike feeling obligated and making any fixed commitments worries them.

The shade and tone of yellow in the aura will help you decide what is relevant, the bright positive shades reflecting the positive, in power attributes and the darker, sludgy shades representing the negative possibilities and areas where attention might be placed, in order to resolve those issues.

Sensitivity

The Yellow Personality has a keen intellect and a radiant personality and they can pick up information from all sorts of sources. They are like a beacon that gives out yet can absorb in too. They don't tend to question where that information comes from, they are open to receive information and people around them may often wonder, "Just how did they know that?"

They may not notice that they are almost too sensitive and can soon get overloaded by people and environments, as it is not always obvious as to what is causing them to feel this way. It won't be just one scenario or one cause, it's because they are absorbing in a lot more of what is around them than some other colors. This is where some awareness of energy work can really help, as they can learn to work with and better manage or protect their energy.

They have an artistic flair which is light and creative. They create because they get pleasure from it, fun will always be involved and important to them. Yet they are also great thinkers and can love philosophical thought and will be interested in concepts that stretch their minds, always with a sense of enjoyment, nothing to dampen their spirit or drag them down.

Yellows tend to be active, on the go and have an abundance of energy, when they are in power. They are not very good at sitting still. You might even notice that when they *are* sat down, they will move their hands or feet quite a lot, they may fiddle with cutlery, napkins or just be very expressive with their hands and body language in general.

They may be writers and authors, even artists as they express themselves with their hands, this can follow through into their work life. They are found in many careers as they are very versatile. It depends on their individual strengths; they may be drawn to creative careers or even philosophical and ideas orientated professions. They make great healers as they are so sensitive to energies and their hands are well tuned instruments.

It's important for Yellows to be able to release the energy they absorb and be able to express themselves as they can become quickly agitated, this agitation is often best expressed through physical movement for them, literally expelling it from their energy system.

Being such an expressive and radiant type, it's usually easy to see exactly how a Yellow is feeling, their body language is usually very obvious and is real; they don't try to hide things. If they are sad you will see it, you will feel they are deflated. An easy way to remember this is to imagine a dog like the Golden Retriever; they can be up and about, bounding around with their tail wagging or they may be curled up in their bed, head down, away from the world. As they are so tuned to energy, their body doesn't lie, it can only express how they are feeling and what is truly going on.

It's important to remember, many of the attributes I have mentioned here are the positive aspects of a Yellow Personality in power. If something affects that power, consider the negative possibilities. For example out of power they may lack any energy or motivation, their get up and go has got up and gone. Just as the words we use can reflect what's going on internally, so does our energy and the way that is expressed.

Being so intimately connected with energy and feeling good, this color will go great lengths to avoid anything that might detract from that. They will try as hard as they can to avoid discomfort and this can leave the door open to put up with people and situations far longer than actually would be good for them.

Out of power, they might stay in an uninspiring job or a bad relationship, which of course just eats into their energy reserves more and more so they can become chronically depleted on all sorts of levels. Then it is all too easy to find quick fixes and miracle cures, getting involved in various distractions and affairs, which only increase the negative cycle.

Yellow Relationships

These are alert and active people on many levels. They like an easy life and don't like heavy commitments in any form. So relationships can be a challenge. They are very sexual and love pleasure but if a relationship restricts them too much, they may just move on. This could lead to a pattern of surface relationships. The fear of commitment being their major concern; they would sooner move away from that possibility, than risk being in love altogether. They may even decide that they don't need a relationship, as it seems to cause more trouble than they deem it is worth.

Yet if you do manage to have a relationship with a Yellow, they can be great partners, very caring and sensitive. Their challenge is the tendency to drop their boundaries in relationships to the extent that they can become depleted and easily feel drained. They need a partner who understands the Yellow traits and who will feed their energy, as a positive Yellow is an abundant and amazing partner to have, who will continually pour energy into the relationship.

They also have a wonderful flirtatious nature and their sexual encounters are felt by their whole body and being. In power they have a visceral understanding of the balance between mind, body and spirit.

Keywords for the Yellow Personality

- Bright
- Sunshine
- Radiant
- Happy
- Energetic
- Humor
- Intelligent
- Sensitive

7 THE GREEN AURA PERSONALITY

The Green Personality is the eternal diplomat; they love harmony and balance and are generally peaceful people. They love a sense of balance and harmony to their relationships, their home, and their wider environment too.

This sense of balance permeates everything in their life, it will be a core value and very important to them. Where some color types might be motivated by sex or money, Greens will evaluate situations and scenarios and be more motivated by what will give them the best sense of balance and harmony. This evaluation process may not be noticeable by others, but Greens will automatically consider how things will make them feel and will accept or decline invitations and opportunities on that 'feeling' basis.

These people have a strong connection with nature and will usually live very close to the countryside, lakes, rivers or the seaside. They know on a visceral level that being outdoors is so good for them; they can almost physically feel their batteries being recharged. It's less about being an optional extra; it is a real necessity for them.

The heart is the organ and area this color primarily relates to. These people determine their lives by how they feel, and they are very honest in evaluating their feelings and emotions. They don't need an object, house or person to look a particular way, what they need is to know that when they look at that object, house or person that they feel good and have a sense of contentment and satisfaction. This cannot be faked. Greens don't want to lie to themselves, nor others, neither do they want a superficial life.

Sometimes people will be shocked at just how open and honest Greens can be and it can seem that they just don't make sense. For example when they are living their lives in balance, Greens need very little to make them happy, they are very content when they are living in line with their heart and their feelings. They don't need a bigger home just because their friends have moved, if they love their home, they love their home, it's as simple as that.

At the same time though, they are not content to just make do, or live below their means. They have their own standards which tend to be relatively high and they like nice things and order, they have an organic sense of abundance about life in general. They usually enjoy a good standard of living, particularly for the things that are important to them.

Abundance

Greens don't pursue success or money, yet seem to somehow magnetically attract all that they need and require. Driven by the heart and a sense for contentment they don't find satisfaction in scrimping and saving, they prefer the middle road of living within their means, whilst enjoying what life has to offer; appreciating the nice things of life without being overtaken by a need to possess them all.

These people tend to make great, loyal friends. They have a profound understanding and acceptance of what it means to be human, the foibles, the potentials, the trials and tribulations. They comprehend the natural rhythms and cycles of life, they understand life moves on, just as the seasons of the year unfold and that we all are ultimately governed by such things. They are not frightened of change but neither do they race ahead trying to instigate it, sometimes they can be a little too laid back and can decide to take life a little too easily, relying on the energy and resources of others.

They seem to spot patterns quickly and have a way of coming up with solutions to problems, they don't get bogged down by the minutiae; they evaluate the whole problem and see the bigger picture and the resulting solution as a natural evolution to the current situation.

The Green Aura denotes someone who is mentally alert and astute; they have a keen intellect and like to use it. They like setting goals and are great at organizing ideas and people but they may not have the impetus to always follow through on those ideas. The energy required for such things can soon drain them and deprive them of their sense of balance. They make great managers and communicators, perfectly describing their processes and projects but not wanting to necessarily be the one to see that project through to fruition.

These are sense based people; they also have a good degree of common sense and practicality. They are very kinesthetic, touch and grounding is very apparent to them.

They have a good connection between their mind and body and they will express their thoughts often through their body, very visibly. They need to feel free to express their emotions otherwise they can feel very restricted and uncomfortable, eventually becoming weakened or ill if they don't.

They can often shock the people close to them by such expressions, as their reactions can be very quick, if they are cross, they will raise their voice straight away, if they are upset, you'll see the tears form very quickly too. They live by their feelings, they don't think about them first. Their bodies understand that the expression is a necessary release and that the sooner the release, the sooner the sense of balance is likely to return. They really don't like the feel and taste of unexpressed emotions or thoughts.

They know that stored words of hurt and resentment can turn very sour and become much worse, they understand that holding on to such emotions also doesn't feel good in their physical system. They have a physical intelligence and awareness of how things feel in their body which is their barometer for discerning life. Much as we might taste a rotten apple and spit it out, that's how a Green can feel about words, thoughts and feelings, their internal sensations and representations can be that obvious and apparent to them.

Greens can have quite high expectations of themselves and of life in general, especially when it comes to money and relationships as these areas are so fundamental to their enjoyment and maintaining that sense of harmony and satisfaction.

They may not be over ambitious but they do want an easy going life, they don't want manic schedules or high stress living. They want a good income but they won't tolerate stringent deadlines and stressful work conditions for long. They like their independence and will like being their own boss. In a relationship they will need space and will enjoy a partner that compliments them rather than challenges them. Even with their own children, if they threaten their sense of peace and harmony, they would find that hard to deal with.

These people make great talkers; they find talking very therapeutic. They can be extremely charismatic and almost magnetic as a speaker. People are naturally drawn to them. They make great teachers as they tend to communicate from the heart. They talk about what they love and like other people to feel good too. They are compassionate and level headed souls, wanting peace and harmony for everybody.

For hobbies these people enjoy being outside, they tend to enjoy gardening, walking the dog, being with horses, possibly swimming in a natural environment. They have a natural affinity with animals and nature and often like to work with one or both within their profession.

When they are out of balance Greens can cut themselves off. Where as they normally like to be around people and communicating is something they love to do, they can become disempowered and then withdraw from people and close themselves off to communication.

Consequently as they shut themselves away, they deprive themselves of their own energy feeds from the environment and from expressing their true nature with people. Then all too quickly, they can find that their life has no substance or meaning anymore. They wonder what their purpose is and can't seem to find it and then give up the struggle to look for it. Depression can seem to envelop them.

Some Greens, turn away from people altogether and give their attention to animals and to nature, they may move to a more secluded location and spend a great deal of time with animals or alone. This can seem a safer alternative to dealing with and confronting daily life, particularly where close relationships are involved.

The risk of loving someone can seem such a threat to the status quo and their sense of peace that they can decide to abstain altogether. Opening themselves up to love and feeling vulnerable can seem a price that they may not be willing to pay. It is important for Greens to understand that to enjoy their sense of power, they need to grow; to feel the flow of love and the gift of relationships is part of our natural evolution and growth, shutting themselves away is just a form of stagnation, fine for the short term as a means of initial recovery and recuperation but not as a long term life choice or pattern.

Greens in power love relationships, they love talking about them, they want everyone to be happy in love and they like to know that everyone has someone to love and care for. In a relationship themselves, they will often be very open and will share their private thoughts and feelings. Sometimes this might not be always what their partner wants to hear. Strangely though it can be quite hard for Greens to make a really deep connection, it can sometimes feel like nobody really 'gets' them.

Greens enjoy intimate relationships; sex for them confirms their sense of aliveness. They appreciate it as being a physical expression of love. They have a natural and organic appreciation of this vital and intimate part of being human.

When they are out of balance, Greens will also try to avoid confronting people or situations. They won't get too involved; they will stay on the periphery, so it might seem they are superficial or disinterested. A sense of passivity can pervade their entire being, a lethargy to living almost. It's like their energy is diminishing, their life force and vitality is in a state of atrophy not growth and it will show in every area of life. Whereas in power they exude life, vitality and abundance in everything they do, out of power they start to disappear, they become a shadow of who they truly are.

A way to re-establish their power and connection is to get involved with a cause or charity, no matter how simple, to see and immerse themselves in genuine, innocent kindness from one person to another. Kindness opens the door to love, seeing and being around simple acts of kindness will remind their heart, what it is that feeds it and how good it feels to give and receive love. Part of what feeds Greens on a spiritual and energetic level is the human interaction with life itself, how we each need the other and how we are all connected to nature and made from the same stuff.

In their career, they will be perceived as friendly and helpful, well liked by people. They may not be the hardest worker and they may not be obviously ambitious or goal driven though. It's not money as such that motivates them, it's less about accumulating wealth as having enough money to enjoy life and do all the things they want to do.

Greens are natural healers and as communication comes so well to these people, they will often be teachers or therapists. Some will be drawn to directly working with nature such as gardeners, vets or something agriculturally based. In the office environment they will often be secretaries or assistants; using their organizational skills to assist other people, without having to be out at the front as the leader.

Deep Green in the Aura

Green in the aura is a bit like its opposite color in the color wheel; red. In that it has a deeper shade which can show slightly different characteristics and traits. In fact they absorb and display many Red characteristics whilst they still embody all of the Bright Green traits and they can take them to an ever deeper level.

People with a deeper shade of green in the aura are intelligent, full of vitality and enjoy a degree of luxury and abundance in their life. Everything about them oozes a sense of wealth and prosperity. They like the luxuries in life and would love it if everyone could live in a world of plenty, experiencing all the very best that life has to offer.

This shade of green is ambitious and can be found in businesses and careers dealing with material assets and wealth. They love careers and past times that will stimulate their mental capacity and are not the sort to suffer fools easily.

When they speak, they can be very intense and powerful people and are very charismatic, often impressing the people around them or the audience they are addressing. There is a sense of commanding impressiveness about this personality, they come across as if they know a better way - and they often do.

Although of course, if out of power this can quickly result in an attitude of superiority, sometimes even being aggressive and impatient. They can be very quick to judge people and can easily dismiss people if they don't meet up to their own high standards and expectations.

Deep Greens have the will power of an ox and as such can be stubborn at times. These are strong characters, perfectionists by nature. They expect the best and this can sometimes cause stress and pressure for the people around them as second best is not an option they would choose to accept or tolerate.

This makes them brilliant event organizers, coordinating teams, managing projects as they will strive for the very best outcome. They can think on their feet and always seem to have a can do attitude that can deal with any issues as they arise.

Deep Greens can often be found amongst the self employed as they like to do things for themselves and don't want to jump to someone else's tune. They are great givers of advice and will always have an answer for a problem.

They like to delegate tasks and can be found in high salaried positions with a degree of scope and status about them too. They like prestige and embody all the positive attributes well. A good way of thinking about them is to imagine they were Royalty, having an air of presence, abundant growth and luxury.

These people are attractive in nature and looks, they seem to draw people in, they are magnetic and will usually have a circle of admirers or followers. Strangely though, they can struggle somewhat when it comes to making deep, intimate bonds, particularly in their personal relationships.

This is often because they find it hard to truly accept people, being Green they are not good at masking over things and they can't pretend they haven't noticed a potential partner's bad habits or foibles. Of course their high standards and expectations can also make it difficult to accept a mate. If the other person is not so full of drive, ambition and energy as them, they can soon become bored and will want to move on.

They like to share an intellectual balance with their partners and will often choose someone in a similar or complementing profession, as they like to talk, and talking shop provides them with stimulation and enjoyment. They prefer discussions with depth, rather than superficial niceties and nonsense.

Sex is less of a driving force with Deep Greens but when they connect with someone, sex can be a very deep experience, on a physical as well as an emotional level for them. Out of power they can disconnect from their emotions and the close intimacy between them and their partner may suffer, so that sex becomes a purely physical act to be enjoyed for what it is in the moment, rather than what it represents to the relationship as a whole.

It's almost as if they have to be impressed by their partner, they need to be someone they can look up to, without feeling jealous of. They thrive with a partner who stimulates them but doesn't challenge them and certainly doesn't disappoint them. They thrive with an equally strong partner.

When they do find a partner they can love however, they are incredibly loyal and will formulate a strong and lasting bond; soul mates in every way.

Keywords for the Green Personality:

- Abundance
- Mind and body balance
- Good communicators
- Money
- Balance
- Nature
- Intelligent
- Honest
- Heart Centered
- Love & Relationships

8 THE BLUE AURA PERSONALITY TYPE

People with a Blue Aura, tend to be the care givers, whether naturally as parents or as a profession, they can be found as nurses and doctors, healers and therapists, as well as in professions to do with legality and honesty, such as the police or judicial system.

This is the color of authority, so if they are not in authority and the color is diminished it is a sign they need to take authority now. In fact with this color you will often come across the extremes: a person who communicates well and is in a position of authority if the color is strong. And if they are out of balance and the color is weaker, you'll probably find a quiet soul who has been the subject of bullying or abuse.

On the whole, I have noticed that I have come across more washed out Blues than vibrant ones. It is not always easy to stand up and say what we really feel and mean and keeping quiet to keep the peace can become a life motto for some.

A lot of the aspects I cover here reflect the more disempowered state, so remember if you feel the shade or tone of blue is strong and vibrant, you would be reading for an assertive, authentic person, in power.

These are honest souls that care about right doing and other people. They are usually quite emotionally moved people and have a naturally kind and giving nature. Unfortunately this can also make them vulnerable, gullible and at some point becoming the victim or martyr in a situation. As with all colors, the potential for extremes exists.

Blues can be the introverts in the spectrum; they are friendly, innocent and loving souls. They love to help others and be of service. They can be very attentive to the needs and wants of other people, especially those they see as being at a disadvantage, the elderly, the very young or the oppressed.

Although they are far from stupid and have a well developed emotional intelligence, especially for other people, they don't seek out intellectual conversations and debate. They can find such situations intimidating and challenging.

They thrive by using their feelings and their intuition based senses, they are not as impressed by facts and figures, more so by deeds and circumstances. Their intelligence has a warm wisdom about it, a caring and encompassing attitude that values how people feel and their sense of truth and justice runs deep within their veins. They seem to instinctively know, just what people need and are able to offer and provide great comfort. These are the healers and nurturers of our world.

When out of power their emotional aptitude can overwhelm their senses and they can lose focus and energy very quickly. It can be as if someone has pulled a plug on their world and they can feel totally disorientated and unsure of what to do. Being so used to helping others they may not be quite so quick to ask for anything for themselves, or even think that they are worthy of someone else's time and attention.

Communication & Authenticity

Blue is the color of communication and Blues communicate in a variety of ways. They can experience very deep feelings which they may express verbally or through art or writing. At times of low energy or disempowerment it can be very therapeutic for blues to write down their story, or to journal and keep a diary, so that they can write their thoughts and feelings out of their system and down onto paper.

Otherwise they can become laden down, feeling lethargic and heavy, a bit like a sponge that has absorbed the maximum amount of water. This saturation point can reveal itself as melancholy or bouts of depression and hopelessness; they can certainly suffer from not being able to see a clear way out of their predicament.

Caring

Mothers often display blue in their aura, caring and nurturing for their children. It's as if this color wants to scoop the world up in its arms and make everyone safe and secure. Blues are good with the sick and needy; they take the time and patience to care. It's almost as if they would devote their life to others, they are very accepting and kind hearted people.

Consequently they are well liked and will have a wide circle of friends, although it may transpire that the Blue is the primary giver. They are also very quick to forgive and this can result in them being taken advantage of and is one area for them to look out for.

Blues can be moved to tears easily and will show their emotions at the drop of a hat, which can be unnerving for some of the other color types. This sensitivity is part of what makes them so good for other people as they really appreciate emotions and feelings, they know how it feels to be hurt and they want to stop the pain as soon as possible.

These people like to stick to the rules and won't push boundaries; they seek a peaceful, quiet life. Often they will even have a very quiet voice or a generally submissive nature and attitude to life. They can regularly feel helpless and may even use such words, they have an attitude that there is nothing that can be done and that it is not for them to challenge things. In other words, when out of sorts, they don't like to take authority and can often hand over their own authority to family members or partners.

This can happen to such an extent that they may be regularly bullied, harassed or even abused by the people around them. They have real problems with being able to say No effectively. They don't want to upset other people or let them down in any way. Consequently they may suffer from a lack of boundaries and take on too much responsibility.

Blues can be the shy and retiring types, they will prefer to hold back rather than stand up and be counted or noticed, unless of course someone else is hurt or in danger, then they are motivated by the desire to save and rescue.

Out of power it's as if they feel they have to be doing something in order to be loved.

Their whole life is primarily focused on other people; their challenge is to remember their own life and self love and respect. It would be all too easy for them to dedicate their life to one of caring or service, only to realize that they had not experienced much of life for themselves and that they never had chance to grow as a person. Then bitterness and sourness can set in.

Relationships

In an ideal world Blues would marry for life, they make wonderful partners as they are so supportive and caring. However as with most things, too much of a good thing, can turn out to be not so good after all.

Out of power they can be suffocating to be around, they can also become very manipulative, to try and create situations where their love is needed, keeping themselves and their partner trapped in a vicious cycle of co dependency. Love and care becomes a trade off situation, if you do this for me, then I will do that for you. Life and love become very conditional.

A lack of self confidence can be a very Blue trait and they can blame themselves for all sorts of things. They can become swamped by self doubt and self pity. They will hold on to the one negative comment they heard and soon forget the five good ones. It's as if they're tuned in for sadness and despair when they are out of power.

Blues need to be aware of what is good for them and what feeds their energy. They also need to know they have an absolute right to the good things in life too; they are not put on this earth only to serve others. They have to learn to include themselves in their loving and caring nature. It is very common to see a disempowered blue and it will often link to their voice and the throat chakra, as this energy center is all about speaking your truth and living in alignment with your true self. Your true self is never a disempowered representation; it is the full, vibrant, empowered and enlivened version of you.

Blues are very family orientated and will often be the one that holds the family together and keeps everyone in touch. They naturally make arrangements for family days out or will always remember birthdays and anniversaries. They like to send and receive letters and cards. They also like to be appreciated for what they do, even if they don't directly ask for it. They are loyal types, who when praised and recognized will remain loyal forever.

Blues are not always the most light hearted of people to be around. They can feel that life has dealt them a hard blow, that nothing can be done about it, and they just have to accept the cards that have been dealt. So although they can be very supportive, it's as if they need someone to rescue or a cause to suffer for in order to feel alive. They are not motivated by improving their own life or situation, but they would do it for someone else. This is a bit like a parent living their dreams through their children.

It's a constant game of balance for all of us, regardless of which color you might be. But the Blues in particular need reminding to look after themselves and keep themselves in power as when they slip out of it, they can become very draining to be around and soon turn into energy vampires.

Which is so far from who they are in power and who they want to be; the nurses and caregivers, the nurturers of the color spectrum.

Think of the Blue Personality as the mother figure, how many mothers do you know who when asked how they are will always say, " Oh I'm fine", almost as a knee jerk response when in truth they need some TLC too. In fact the mother is a good analogy as she can be the wonderful nurse, the care giver but also consider how many people have a bad relationship with their mother and all those negative attributes that can go along with that character, the manipulative controlling figure. There are positive and negative aspects to every character trait and so it is with every color.

Blues relate very much to the word harmony and sound, the organs of communication are very important to this color type. The ears and eyes, throat all correspond to this aura color and the Throat Chakra.

In a relationship the physical act of sex and love making is of less importance than finding a true mate and companionship. They can seem to enjoy cuddling and kissing more. They want a mate for life and as a result will stay in an unhealthy relationship much longer than is good for them. In fact they can find it almost impossible to let go. Indeed, letting go is not something they tend to be good at generally. They can hold on to hurt and resentment and out of power will find forgiveness to any degree, very difficult if not impossible.

Blues are often drawn to find out more about our spiritual nature and will enjoy learning about the different disciplines. They don't need much convincing when it comes to ethereal subjects and psychic phenomena, which again is an area where they can be easily led or deceived.

Money is no great motivator for these people, they are conservative by their nature and know that money is required but it will not take the place of the importance of people in their lives.

They can be indecisive and will go with the majority vote in most instances.

They are not that keen on physical prowess or activity and can be prone to putting weight on and even hoarding or amassing clutter in their lives generally.

In their most positive aspect Blues are great orators and entertainers, working in television or radio, where they have a profession in presenting, speaking and talking. Often this though is more to do with entertainment rather than opening up about themselves personally. It's almost as if they have a perfect aspect to their persona for presenting and expression, yet still retain a very private and almost withdrawn or introverted aspect to their own personal life and journey.

A challenge for Blues can be to learn to take their own counsel, they will ask questions and seek guidance from others, finding out how they would tackle a problem, when the one person they don't ask or listen to is their own innate inner wisdom and guidance. It can be as if their ears are so tuned on to external listening and the voices of others that they forget to stop and listen to themselves. If they could find a way to center themselves and get still long enough, they would hear that quiet voice within them that will always guide them in the right direction.

Keywords for the Blue Personality

- Sincere
- Communicative/ Quiet
- Carer, Nurse
- Mother
- Nurture
- Sensitive
- Harmony
- Authority/Taken Advantage Of

9 THE INDIGO AURA

The Indigo Personality is a nice person to be around. They have an air of authenticity and open honesty about them. They are aware of the potential and beauty of consciousness, the human consciousness as well as the higher consciousness.

They will usually have a spiritual outlook on life and humanity as a whole. It's as if they were born knowing. The saying an 'old head on young shoulders' fits with these people very much. They would have been the sort of child that just knew what was expected of them, or how things worked.

The trouble can be sometimes in Indigo children that they can make the adults around them uncomfortable, especially those who try to make them conform in some way - such as teachers and authority figures. It's as if Indigos know the rules and they don't want or need to be continually reminded or restrained by them.

Out of power this can lead to behavioral problems and they will feel like nobody really understands them. My favorite saying was; "It's as if I've been dropped off in a foreign land by mistake", because sometimes it can feel like they are talking a different language and that they care and appreciate things on such a deep and expansive level that it can be hard to put across in words, which then becomes a frustration. Although the written word can be beautiful, it still does not quite do justice to the way the Indigos feel, see and interpret their world.

These people are deep thinkers and feelers, even if it is not always obvious. They can seem to blend in on the surface but really, they tend to always feel like they're the square peg trying to fit in a round whole. That is until they realize that if they only stopped trying to fit, the world around them would mold itself perfectly to fit around *them*.

Their love of authenticity runs deep within their veins, they act in line with their values and ideals and like the people around them and whom they count as friends to act congruently with their nature too. They much rather someone admit to wrong doing and faults, rather than hide them or sweep them away in some kind of distraction. They need to look in the eyes of their partner and know that they would speak the truth, even if it was a painful truth, as to Indigos a lie hurts so much more. This is of course, an attribute, when they are in power and feeling good, consider how that might be reversed and you will get a notion of what might be happening for them if they are out of sorts.

Indigos have a badge of honor and decency about them, which coupled with strength and a reserve of courage that embodies them, they will not be easily bent or persuaded by others and they do not want to be told how to live or be.

Their sense of fairness and justice and right doing guides them throughout life and it can be hard for them to have to slow down and listen to mundane rules and regulations that hardly seem worthy of mentioning as they have already taken them as being part of their natural order of things.

These lovely people know there is so much more to us than meets the eye; they know we don't stop existing where our skin ends, even if they can't always express it. They can have long periods of time where they are angry or frustrated by life. Imagine growing up as an aware child, knowing the world and the universe is an amazing place, connecting all forms of life, yet not having the words to express or explore that. Then consider what might happen if your parents and the people around you, during your formative years are not so aware, or are shut off completely or maybe have dysfunctional lives in one form or another. It is easy to see how confusions and disorientation might set in. What they are 'taught' can be at direct odds with what they 'know'.

It's almost as if they were born into a world knowing, then were 'educated' and taught that things were not that way and that to survive they have had to conform to a way of being and living that goes against everything they somehow know or feel in their heart. There is then this internal battle between head and heart: between knowing and feeling.

It's like their childhood and youth are spent learning a life that is restrictive and alien to them but **that** society has words and language and formats that everyone else, certainly those in authority seem to be abiding to and expounding. Then at some point, usually in their adult life, they will have an awakening of some kind that will shake them to their core and they realize that in their innocence, what they knew and felt *was* right all along.

Knowing that everything and everyone is connected they will have a humanitarian approach and will not knowingly want to harm or destroy anything. They will often have a close affinity with animals and nature; it is an extension of their consciousness rather than being something separate from it.

These people are guided by how they feel in their heart and won't need statistics to prove something that they intuitively feel is right.

In times gone by, they would be found in spiritual professions or religious groups as that will have been the only obvious way to practice their devotion and faith. It's not that they prefer any specific religion but they have always had an awareness of something bigger than themselves, it's just the language that governs our world may not have been there before, only in the realm of spiritual traditions.

Indigos can be easily misunderstood and misinterpreted. They can seem a little introverted at times or even eccentric and a little weird for the more conventional amongst us. Yet in their flow, they are bright and very inspirational to be around. They have a sense of integrity about them but they won't flaunt themselves or their beliefs. It's almost as if their wisdom and beliefs are private things, yet they want everyone to know and experience them too.

Indigos can be very creative and can seemingly tap into thin air and get inspired ideas and suggestions, it's as if they open their mouth and great stuff just seems to pour out.

They seem to just 'get' spirituality and all the many forms of discipline and practice or interest within it. They just know each tradition is another form of expressing what they feel to be true; they may get drawn to individual aspects for a while, especially if they are re-awakening to their true nature after a period of having been 'dumbed down' in normal, conventional life.

Soon though, they realize that spirit is a language that has many dialects and they understand that no particular one is any more or less right than the other. It's almost at times that they are looking for THE way, but the Indigo's challenge is to find and create THEIR way, then all paths lead to happiness and fulfillment and living the life of integrity and authenticity that they love and need. Embracing their true nature gives everyone else permission to do the same.

As far as their physical body goes they can be very sensitive, it's as if their body is an antenna for anything that is bad for them. They can be very sensitive to food additives, alcohol and even to air conditioning and electromagnetic fields.

In power they will be aware of the need to nurture their body rather than abuse or ignore it, they will understand it is the means by which they experience life and will consider their diet and exercise more carefully. They love to walk, maybe jogging but they are not usually keen on excessively hard workouts. They love meditative practices and spiritual exercises.

Indigos make great artists, writers, film makers, imagery in general is important to them. They may be drawn to dance as they like to have fun in the body they are in and all the joys that come with being human.

They are naturally intuitive and will often be drawn to working with energy or spirit in some way, either by channeling directly or using one of the many tools provided in the 'alternative arena' or in a more formal religious or spiritual capacity.

These are compassionate and accepting souls. It's as if they've had a dialogue with angels before they came here and therefore anything that goes against the highest good of themselves and others would contradict what they learnt from that discussion.

The major struggle for Indigos is to live life as they know internally it should be. If they were not supported or nurtured to follow their own path they might have grown up with a false message of having to conform and that they were somehow 'wrong'. They can now appear as very confused and disorientated adults, with a lot of tension and angst and often a string of misdemeanors to their name.

For some of them, it's as if they had to get 'out of their head' as everyone around them seemed to be telling them one thing, whilst usually doing another and all of that contradicting what they felt inside. The way to stop that internal confusion may have been to create external confusion, becoming what people told them they would, as they had no other obvious way of being. If they didn't choose the 'create chaos' route then they may have plumped for the quiet and more submissive route, trying to conform and hide in some way.

Thankfully now, times are such that society is much more accepting and embracing. Even if there are no concrete answers, their perceptions are not ridiculed or persecuted. Now is the time for them to carve their life in their own image and to come alive. To light the way, as in power these people are magnets for lost souls and they hold the torch to light the way with such compassion and empathy.

In power it's as if they have angel wings themselves. Not in a light and fluffy sense but in the sense that the genuine sincerity and integrity of their heart knows only compassion for the spirit and soul. They understand what it means to be human and they also will not allow that to be an excuse anymore to deviate from who they truly are. To walk the spiritual path is not an easy ride and at times requires hobnail boots and a warrior attitude as well as a pair of angel wings but their heart will always be true.

As far as their personal life and relationships go, Indigos can embody both male and female aspects to their psyche. Sometimes male Indigos can have a few female characteristics or traits, we'd say today that they are in touch with their feminine side. The female Indigo tends to be able to turn her hand to most things and will often be very practical too.

Their male and female energies are both strong and it can be that they are less bothered by relationships. They won't feel a *need* for one but when they do find a true mate they make great lovers and partners.

Indigos view sex as a physical merging of their spiritual energies. They need support and understanding; they want to look in their partners' eyes and see love at the same time as feeling it through their heart. It's a reminder of the love that they recognize from that they tasted of the universe itself and it becomes tangible to them through their partner.

In their career choice, Indigos need to be able to be themselves and work in environments and in a way that suits them. They will want a good degree of flexibility and independence and they will always prefer honest professions and dealings over anything unscrupulous or misleading.

Of all the personality types, these people really do need to consider their environment - not just at work or at home but in everything. Being very sensitive, the wrong environment can be very destructive to them. This can be on a physical, mental, emotional or spiritual level and the awareness of all of these different aspects of themselves are plates that they will always have to keep spinning and be aware of, to enjoy life to the full. If they get their environments right and create spaces and daily habits for themselves that are conducive to their nature and psyche they will shine and flourish like never before.

The Indigo needs strong, nurturing foundations in place to be able to stand up, be seen, be noticed and do what they came here to do. They have leadership qualities that need to be expressed - they may have kept quiet because of fear of ridicule and not being accepted. And it can seem that their life is full of contradictions. If they've had a lifetime of being told to conform or be quiet and behave, to stand up and take the lead can seem a daunting task, yet it is one they were made for and will do so well.

Keywords for the Indigo

- Sensitive
- Intuitive
- Inner knowing
- May have been misunderstood or in trouble
- Considerate
- Spiritual/Meditative

10 THE VIOLET AURA

People with a Violet Aura can be one of the most complex auras to read, as in full strength and power they seem to embody the positive aspects of the other colors in the spectrum, equally when they are out of power or blocked they can encounter all of the more negative aspects.

They can be charismatic and dynamic leaders, filled with innovative and visionary ideas and ideals. They want the world to be a better place and seem to know how it can be done. They merge ideas and action and can be very powerful and exciting to be around.

Violets will often talk about the 'bigger picture' and the 'end game'. They can see a better way. They can visualize easily and will come up with new ways of doing things and have some truly inspired ideas. They can pluck ideas from the ether and can then follow it through to make it a reality. They won't get bogged down in details and facts, if they can see it clearly in their minds eye and feel it is true in their heart; which is all the confirmation and fuel they require.

Other people around them can find Violets annoying and baffling as they seem to work the world under their own terms, normal rules do not apply to these types and annoyingly they are usually right.

These are the inventors and inspirers of the color spectrum. They are also great thinkers, they will like theories and will be quite philosophical about life. They will get to the root cause that might be underlying any problems or issues. They will look further than the surface, they won't stop at the symptom, and they will want to get to the root of things.

Being a beautiful merging of red and blue they need to embrace the qualities and traits of both colors. They are sensitive yet strong, supportive yet active, they are gentle yet passionate. As you can see there is a lot of scope for ups and downs or what seems like behavior swings, but Violets are all of these things.

Once they and the people around them understand this, it can make for a much smoother experience for all. Until we know the aspects of our personality and of those around us, how can we truly accept them and create situations and circumstances where our best aspects can shine? Violets especially need to know what does and doesn't work for them as they can confuse themselves with what they sense and feel.

Violets are fascinated by other people and by life itself. They can be very charismatic and have a magnetic personality that draws you in. They also have an emotional intelligence and awareness that makes them nice people to be around and have within your circle of friends. They don't stop at compassion and kindness; they can see a way out and want the best for everyone.

In their vibrant power they can be magical, in touch with the grounded beauty of our physical world and also their minds stretch into the ethereal realms of possibility and bring that wonder down to earth too.

Out of balance or power, they can easily seem to have drifted off a little too far and may be perceived as a little too weird or having lost the plot entirely. This can be because they have found the pull of their spiritual nature and what they experience there as a much more attractive prospect than dealing with what appears to be the mundane experiences of our modern day life and all the strife and troubles that can bring.

These people usually are very fond of music, if they don't play an instrument, music will be an important part of their life. Music and sound can transport them to a better place in their mind and they can get a real physical sensation of bliss and euphoria from particular beats and rhythms. Music and sound can be particularly healing for them.

Connected

Violets tend to need a lot of space, that is physically and mentally. They are independent people not afraid of their own company and they need space around them. They can feel hemmed in and restricted in large towns and cities and you may even see them physically cringe or seem to diminish in size when they have to visit one. They will be impatient to get out and away.

They do their best thinking away from the melee of life. They have an almost tangible connection to the universal energy and are very aware of anything that gets in the way of that. The towns and cities have too much white noise as it were; so much so, that it feels like it adversely interrupts their frequency and connection.

People can think that Violets are not easy to approach as from the outside they may seem distant or uninterested. Yet on the inside, when people are brave enough to get closer they are warm and sensitive people brimming with passion and empathy. They can be reserved in their initial emotions with people as they have the sensitive nature of Blues and also the passion of Red. This is where they can come across as cold, as their feelings run so deep that when they get hurt, it really hurts and it is hard for them to forget that pain. That cool exterior is their protection to try and prevent that hurt from having the chance to sneak its way in again.

People around them will say this person is calm, confident, self assured and a very strong person, if you asked the same question of the Violet though, they would tell a different story. They would know that the exterior does not always translate to how they feel internally. They can be their own worst enemy and are very strong critics of themselves. They can often be perfectionists and will at some level, usually deep inside, feel unworthy or even guilty of the good things that happen in their life.

Even when something has gone well, they will probably think it could have gone better. It's as if they are painfully aware of their own imperfections and these can be easily used as a means to hold themselves back.

Violets will soon get cross if they can't do something relatively quickly. When learning a new skill if they haven't got a better than average grasp within a couple of lessons, they will not be happy. They have set such high standards of themselves that they would never expect anyone else to ever reach and are often totally unaware of these exacting standards and the effect they might be having on their own experience of life.

Violets need a cause, a reason for being. They will want to achieve something with their life, to make a difference to people. To leave the world a better place than when they entered. Having the energy and dynamism of red this is totally possible for these people.

They have the insight and passion to do a great deal of good to the world we live in. As soon as they recognize this urge though, their next thought is to question their ability to really make a difference and who do they think they are?

They almost feel they should be a bigger and better person before they can really stand up and make that difference. Yet it burns in their energy. This is where they need support and encouragement from the people around them as they are the champions of the cause with the gusto required to get the task done and done well.

Intuitive

One of the toughest tasks for a Violet is to actually listen to and trust their strong intuition. They can have so many great ideas, which genuinely are great that they can find it hard to settle on one and will become disorientated and confused.

This is where they need a strong, caring and supportive partner at home or at work. To nurture all that's good in them, to take their ideas and make them work, whilst not allowing them to get overwhelmed and bogged down. With a Violet there is always another possibility.

Out of power, then Violets might be perceived as arrogant or a little pompous, thinking that they are better than other people and have a right to a bigger slice of the cake than anybody else. They can have a hardened attitude to those less fortunate and be very dismissive of people. If this is allowed to continue and grow then their ego can become very inflated and they will be domineering characters, bullies, wanting to be liked and admired by people and willing to manipulate to get that adoration by any means.

Violets need people and activities that allow them to expand but also that keep them in touch with reality as it is all too easy for them to detach from that.

They have an innate understanding and comprehension of spiritual matters, they see God in everything, they understand it is a universal concept and they are an extension of that. Some kind of spiritual practice will be important to Violets and they will gain a great sense of peace and enjoyment from that connection.

They understand the concept of us being co creators of our own experiences and in power will manifest easily and abundantly. Out of power they may still manifest abundantly but it will more likely be of the chaotic variety. They 'get' that mind and body are just two parts of the same thing and the energy of spirit and emotion are the fuel, the successful merging and directing of which is what creates the things we see around us.

Violets can seem to have such extremes in their character and this is seen even in their social life. They can seem antisocial, even saying that they don't really 'do people', yet when they do get together with others they can enjoy nothing more than a good conversation. Particularly so if it is a one on one conversation that is entertaining, intellectual or philosophical. Mundane social gatherings and idle chit chat don't hold their attention or interest for long; they just can't see the point of that. They would much rather go to a meeting to discuss projects, ideas or business possibilities than the trivialities of life.

It's as if they have to accept and embrace the opposites they have within their character to be able to feel happy with who they are. They can shut themselves off from people and exclude themselves from society all too easily. It is important that they don't become the eternal hermit and they come out every now and then for some light hearted fun. To taste the good things that life has to offer as they can become serious thinkers and loners left to their own devices.

These are kind hearted souls who will always be found helping someone out, often for little or no remuneration. Money is not one of their major motivators. They understand it brings freedom and luxury and is necessary and that in the right hands it can bring many great things to the world. They don't need much for themselves though; they will usually spend it on friends and family before they treat themselves. They are often good with money in that they are not frivolous spenders, nor are they hoarders.

Relationships

In a relationship Violets need someone who really understands them and appreciates them. Much like Indigos, they don't feel the need for relationships and will go without for periods of time. They would rather be on their own than spend years in a bad partnership, they don't need the company as much as they do the real connection.

Sex for Violets is a merging of energies and a delightful experience that transcends the physical act. They are sensitive and intuitive and are very considerate partners when they meet someone with whom they will share their time here on earth. They will often be drawn to tantric practices as they want to experience the merging of consciousness at the point of orgasm and will enjoy the ecstasy of that. It's a deep relationship with a Violet or it's not one at all I'm afraid!

They can demand a lot from their partner as they can be so intense. When they commit, they really commit and their energies and focus will flow towards their mate. These people can merge with their partner to an extent that they can lose their own identity and strength, so both partners need to understand and be aware of that. It's as if they morph into one and may often live and work together too, which can be a great thing but also has its potential pitfalls.

It's hard for Violets to stay present in a relationship at times. They can withdraw into their own space and would find it hard to open up and share to a partner, especially if they felt let down or hurt in some way. They let people in at such a deep level, so deep they almost become one as it were and if something happens that hurts, it hurts deep and they will go straight back to protective mode and close down. This is not necessarily a conscious reaction but if you mention it, they or their partners and families will recognize it.

Love and connection is never superficial with these people and when hurt, it would not be like losing a finger and having the attitude ok let's move on, it would be more like, losing a leg; really rocking their world.

If they should lose their life partner, they may decide that there is no one else for them, they mate for life, heart and soul so will not usually be one for casual encounters and relationships.

Leaders

If only the Violet would realize they are a born leader and step into that role, their life would be so much easier. They need support and encouragement and when they do, they realize that doors seem to magically open for them. They may even say that they have lived a charmed life. That they cope well, things don't really get to them so much and they don't get bogged down by life.

This is the positive result from their ability to keep a distance, to observe life without having to take part in it too much. Their greatest pain will be from the loves they have encountered. It is how they have dealt with these that will determine their holding of power and how they present themselves to the world.

These people are very intelligent, it's like they seem to have it all going for them, the only person that doesn't think so is themselves. There are lots of potential ways to conquer their own particular version of self doubt and when they do, the world is their oyster.

Violets are often found in the acting profession, as entertainers and presenters. They have a dynamic stage presence and people love to be drawn in by their magnetism and charm. They also make great artists, writers, musicians; they love history and philosophy, old subjects as well as new technologies. They are fascinated by our world and retain their curious attitude.

To be happy, Violets need to live life how they feel it should be. Once they have the confidence and self belief they can move on in leaps and bounds and start waking people up to their world vision and a better way for all. They need to express their visions and ideas, to get them out there so they can feel a sense of fulfillment and achievement. They have to drop the small vision they have of themselves and step into the bigger persona they truly are. They will know this as a truth when you speak with them.

Keywords for the Violet Personality

- Leader
- Charismatic
- Authentic
- Magical
- Music
- Passion
- Self doubt
- Visionary
- Innovative & Intuitive

11 THE CRYSTAL AURA

Depending on how and where it shows, white in the aura can show energy being drained away - particularly if it feels more like it's washing out the main core color. It might give you the impression of grey or patchiness, so it requires some close attention, to determine what is really going on.

White as a core color by itself though is a different thing and to be honest is probably not one that you will come across that much. It can sometimes be known as the Crystal Aura.

The White or Crystal Personality is someone, who is not only aware of the greater consciousness and the universal energies but they can actively merge with them and act as a conduit or channel for those energies in some way. That may be by directly communicating as a spiritual channel or by teaching and healing.

White, is not really a color, it is an absence of color and is the result of all of the rainbow colors combined into one beautiful prism. These people love to absorb knowledge, they will never tire of finding out about the world we live in. Their life can be determined by how clear they are about their internal feelings and how much energy they absorb and channel through their system. They will be motivated by their knowledge of the cosmic energies and will thrive on sharing what they know and feel.

They want each one of us to know just how unique and amazing we are and to realise our own potential. This is a kind of transcendent thinking without the need to call it by a particular name or expect it to look a certain way.

These people are often quiet but their mind is active, they are quick minded and intelligent, they will also pay good attention to their intuition and the wisdom that comes from their heart.

Although they want the best for people, and are natural healers, the Crystal Soul, likes time on their own; they actively need and enjoy it. To these people their inner world is as tangible and real as the external one, it is not an either or scenario.

The clearer the channel, the brighter their energy, a bit like a real crystal, if they become bogged down with thought and emotion, this can soon cloud their healing and intuitive abilities. Their whole being is like a big reflection of the energy they're absorbing and channeling; any stuck energy will soon slow the channel and clog the system.

When Crystals are with other people, they can be hard to work out as they seem to morph into a similar resonance to those they are with. They can take on mannerisms, sayings and attitudes of the other color personalities. This is one of the ways that they gain a great rapport with people, many of whom will be drawn and enthralled by the Crystal Personality.

The Crystals that are aware of their abilities and 'calling' will use this to heal themselves and others, in whatever form that takes. Some even seem to take on and step into the energy of the other person, where they then can better determine exactly what needs to be done. Some people might notice an energy drain when they are around Crystals in this kind of mode.

Physically speaking, people with a white aura, can seem a little delicate. They will also like the spaces they live and work in to be conducive and clean, aiding their energy rather than detracting from it. They won't like clutter or feel the need for lots of possessions.

Being extremely conscious of their energy, Crystals will usually be keen to have some kind of energy work in their day, knowing how to keep their channel flowing freely. At the hint of feeling overloaded or clogged, they will want to withdraw and regain a sense of balance. Their energetic body is as tangible as their physical body to these people.

They won't like emotionally or mentally charged atmospheres or stressful ones. Their keywords are peace and tranquility, they are cautious types and peace will always be a stronger motivator than standing out and unnecessary attention.

Out of sorts, these people might suffer from depression and a sense of disorientation. If they get used to not listening to their gut instincts and intuition they can easily get lost and confused, literally but also metaphorically.

Here is where they can also take on other people's characteristics to the extent that they lose themselves and can really struggle to hold on to the thread of who they are and what they came here for.

These people can then suffer from a lack of self confidence as they might feel isolated from the rest of the people around them. To Crystals our spiritual nature and connection is not something they are just interested in or talk about, it is something they feel. It's this strong connection that allows them to spend so much time on their own. It's like they feed on the essence of devotion, the essence of their higher self. The language they use to describe that essence or presence might vary, safe to say though, that it is godlike to them.

Crystal Clear Relationships

In a relationship, it is vital the Crystal be nurtured, understood and given space. They would not usually match so well with Red, Orange or Yellow personalities; as these can be too dynamic, physically, mentally and emotionally. A Green Aura might offer them understanding and a Blue will be willing to care and will feel at ease with their sensitivity. Lavender and Violet personality types can have many of the same characteristics and so might afford them a more peaceful and conducive match.

Keywords for the Crystal Personality:

- Transcendence
- Healing
- Spiritual Channel
- Chameleon
- Meditative
- Teacher/ Spiritual Counselor
- Peace and Tranquility
- Aware of Greater Consciousness and Tapping into that Vibration

12 PINK IN THE AURA

Both green and pink are colors that can be attributed to the heart chakra and both deal with love. For me and what I've seen, Pink is about self love and is connected with our own inner child.

It is a soft and welcoming color, it's like a big, pink, fluffy blanket surrounding and comforting the person. It might indicate some self care, self love and self respect are a part of the person's regime at the moment. A patchy or weak sense of the color might suggest that those things are required.

The inner child is a powerful part of our psyche and I will often dialogue with it directly but to begin with, it is enough to know it exists. If it interests you, I would encourage you to read more about it, if only for your own personal development and growth.

In general there is an innocent childlike feel to this color. If you think how a child can be, you might imagine a lovely, playful soul, all sweetness and light, or you might see an angry toddler having a tantrum! As with all of the colors and all of the attributes there is a light and dark potential, which coincides with the positive and not so positive characteristics.

It's not about one being wrong or right but sometimes if you get an image or sensation of the angry toddler energy, this may relate to either an issue in their childhood or the fact that the person in front of you is being unnecessarily harsh on themselves in some way. This was precisely the case for one lady who came to me for a reading with her friend:

We started the reading in the normal way and as I started to focus on her energy, as crazy as this may sound I saw her inner child pop out and cower behind her, I knew in that instant that, the inner child was afraid of this woman as an adult.

That may not make much sense to some people, but I knew it related to the fact that this lady, as an adult was treating herself harshly. She was being her own toughest critic and so far removed from the innocent, loving child she had been.

I concentrated on the child and dialogued with her in my mind, to find out why she seemed so scared; after all ideally she would reside happily inside the adult body. (The child within us all can hold such magic for us. To me it's as if they are the bridge to our creative excellence and the key holders for that deep sense of happiness and peace we all seek).

As I focused, I soon got an impression of her father, being a strict military man and constantly being moved from place to place, the child was dizzy, disorientated and afraid. She bore the brunt of some harsh treatment. All this was coming from a gentle fractured sense of pink around the woman's ankles and lower legs.

The lady was seated and had her back to me at the time, as I turned, I saw her face was streaked with tears of recognition. She began nodding her head and then relayed the story of her childhood and how now she was indeed being the strict and rigid colonel but to herself; in the very years when she could be truly free and enjoying her days.

I had no idea of such things before I started, I had just learnt to trust that I would see what was relevant and appropriate for the client to know or see.

We discussed her options and she made plans with her friend to make sure she was kinder to herself and would start enjoying her life. She reconnected with that small frightened girl within and promised to now look after her and make her feel safe and loved. It was as if she "became whole that day", was how she later described it to me.

13 BROWN IN THE AURA

Brown in the aura, is often seen in patches, rather than being as a strong core color. It is usually seen with a mix of one or all of red, orange and yellow.

Basically it denotes a practical and grounded personality, someone who will be interested in and motivated by family and their family roots and traditions. They are usually security conscious, wanting to protect and hold on to what they have worked for.

They can put down strong roots and at times those roots in the form of thoughts, can reveal a solid stubbornness in attitude. Think of a large oak tree, with established roots; the things it has relied on for its existence and survival and you get a good idea about the Brown Personality.

These people's minds are active, they are great thinkers and will analyze things before they make a decision or commitment. They are very rational and practical and are great for making sure all the steps are in place and followed; so they make good executors of plans and designs.

They are a great team member to have alongside the more visionary personalities of the color spectrum.

The Brown Personality will focus on the aspect that is important right now and do not need to see the bigger picture, they focus on the job in hand, until that is done and the next job needs to be done.

They may stay in the same location and/or job for many years. They are not great friends with change for change sake. "If it's not broken, don't fix it" will be their motto.

Out of power, this might translate as a fixed stubbornness and a refusal to budge. They can be very skeptical souls and may find a thousand reasons not to do something. Even if they are proven to be wrong on something, they will often remain adamant that they are right.

These people are not usually the type to show their emotions very much, there's an air of solidity about them, rather than frivolity. They may find it difficult to truly relax and slow down as their mind seems to be forever churning over potential pitfalls and concerns.

Browns are usually well respected, as people feel safe in their reliability and honesty, they'll arrive on time and do exactly what they promised to do. They will err on the side of conservatism and cautiousness in just about every area of life.

Relationships

In a relationship, these people are honest, hardworking types, with a strong bond to their family. They are good providers and will enjoy a stable relationship and once committed, they tend to stay committed. They are in it for the long term, no short term whims here!

For careers, Browns prefer solid jobs and workplaces, where they won't be worried about the next pay check. They don't like risks and fluctuations. They can be found in all sorts of professions, from doctors, to computer related careers, electricians and bankers.

Grounded or Sludgy?

Brown in the aura can indicate a grounded person, if however it feels sludgy or clammy in any way it could indicate that the energy is blocked in the region it is showing up.

Keywords for the Brown Aura Personality Type:

- Grounded
- Traditional
- Home and Family
- Stubborn
- Security Conscious

14 CHAKRAS - THE ENERGY CENTERS OF THE AURA

As we covered earlier, there are seven main energy centers, called chakras in the human energy body. There are more but for our purposes here, we'll keep to the main seven.

These run from the bottom of the spine and the Root or Base Chakra, right the way up to the Crown Chakra at the top of the head. These all help to make up the aura and when you want to get more detailed in your readings, you will inevitably delve deeper down into these.

The chakras are not static, they are constantly regulating your energy, 24 hours a day; they are alive and moving. They are taking in and expelling out energy all the time, it's a constant process, just like breathing.

To begin with it is enough to just have a basic idea of what each one relates to; they have emotional, physical, mental and spiritual links to our lives. Indeed the weaker chakra energy is often where an illness will present itself first. This is one area that you can learn more about to better manage your own health and wellbeing. In the resource section you'll find links to my first book on chakra balancing which may be of interest to you and will considerably help your aura readings.

Again, when reading energy, it is not for us to diagnose or worry people. If anything it can be to just confirm that they may be having knee problems right now for example or I will often get a sensation of an old injury or surgery, when I look deeper into the centers.

Here are a few core attributes and associations for each of the chakras:

The Base or Root Chakra

This chakra is located as you might expect at the very bottom of the spine. It is associated with the color red. This energy center is all about the things that allow us to stand up straight and tall in this world, the things that make us strong, confident and physically able to take part in life. It is also a center of manifestation, the physical ability to make things happen; the creative energy to give life to things.

So what sort of things are we talking about here? Well, sex, money, core relationships, home and family as well as things fundamental to life; your overall physical activity and health, your dynamism, your skeleton, your blood.

Physical Health:

The Base or Root Chakra is fundamentally linked to your physical strength and vitality; the life in your body, the blood running through your veins and your ability to adequately function in the world. It relates to your entire skeleton, and particularly the hips, legs and feet. It is about feeling connected and grounded in your physical body and how you experience your life.

Core Relationships:

One of the things that affects how safe and secure we feel is the state of our closest relationships: our intimate partners, our family, as well as the people we socialize and work with. As emotional beings and with emotions being so very powerful, we should never underestimate just how important our relationships are to the smooth running and enjoyment of our lives.

Rifts and tension within the family, the search for birth mothers and fathers, family feuds, all of these can affect our Base Chakra energy.

Safety & Security:

In ancient times, our feelings of safety and security were linked to our ability to stay alive and to find food to eat. We may not be required to hunt for our food these days but our equivalent is all tied up with how we provide for ourselves.

Today that usually means money, so our work life and our ability to earn are implicated here. Without money for food, rent or mortgage payments, we invariably feel threatened.

Fear of failure and feeling inadequate can be Root Chakra issues. So can the eternal push for perfection and setting impossibly high standards.

If there is not enough money coming in and you can't pay the mortgage, that can affect how you feel about life and your own sense of self worth. If your core relationships are unhappy, then that can slow it up too. If your sex life is complicated, non-existent or one of the other extremes, then it will also show up here.

Now that you get a sense of the aspects involved with the Base Chakra, you can no doubt come up with other areas of importance and significance. It's not necessary to try and remember the individual meanings and aspects, far better to remember this energy center is really about our root; our core needs, our instincts and the things we need to survive, not just as an individual but as a race.

Alongside that, sit the mental and emotional basics we need for a sense of safety and security, remember these may be similar for many adults but for children and younger adults, their needs and vital concerns may not be about work, mortgages and landlords, they may be school, college and boyfriends, and about being socially accepted by their peers.

The Sacral Chakra

This chakra is all about creativity and your passion, your desire for things. It is associated with the color orange. Positioned below the navel, governing the internal sex organs and the lower back and belly. This chakra is all about relationships, not just the ones we have with people, but the ones we have with anything and everything, from sex to food, alcohol and drugs.

Creativity & Reproduction

Creativity and reproduction are vital to our survival as a human race and also to our evolution. This force is incredibly powerful; we can create another life - how amazing is that? The vital life force lies behind everything but especially so with our creativity; it can be felt in our wants and desires. Which is a great thing, those desires and wants motivate us to take action, to make change and to create life the way we would like it to be.

But what happens when life doesn't seem to go that way, when things are blocked or our challenges seem to far outweigh our opportunities? This kind of blockage or frustration will show up in this energy center and it can be really quite depleted and stifled. You will get a sense of this as you read this area of the body.

Desire

Orange being a mixture of red and yellow brings attributes of both the neighboring chakra centers. The red adrenaline and instinctual drive with the yellow willpower and control merge into our sacral chakra: an emotional hub of passion, desire and want.

We can desire to be fit and healthy, we can desire a nice home or nice new, shiny car; desire and wanting are things that we feel without too much conscious thought.

We don't make ourselves desire, we just realize we do. Here is where many of us can suffer as we might have been taught that it is wrong to want anything or to have dreams and wishes. That it is selfish or greedy. Take a desire to extremes and it can become an addiction. It's all about balance and the chakras show us that so very clearly.

Emotions

The Sacral Chakra is also our emotional center. Our emotions are what make us human. They are incredibly powerful and can also be trampled upon, abused and neglected, stuffed under a carpet somewhere, only to explode at some later point in a whole variety of ways. Hopefully you are getting a sense of just how vital and powerful this energy center is.

Shock or trauma can often be lodged here in this chakra center as our emotions can take quite a battering at times and knots of tension and stress can sit here which eventually may reveal themselves in a physical way.

Reading this center requires subtlety and compassion as it is so directly connected with our felt emotions and any issue with a strong connection to a past or present situation, will usually reveal itself here.

In a deeper reading it is common for me to gently start describing what I feel about this area for a person and they will be moved to tears; at recognition of someone voicing things that are personal and pertinent to them. So great sensitivity and appropriate disclosure are always required.

Unless you are a trained therapist, avoid trying out any therapy! Keep your readings intentionally accurate but light. However, qualified therapists may like to incorporate aura and energy work into their skill set and current practice to deepen the experience and healing.

The Solar Plexus

This is your power center, the center of your energy reserves; energy comes in and goes out from here. This is about your power, your sense of self worth and inner strength.

It is linked with your will and your willpower. It links with your boundaries (or lack of them). It's about control and is a psychic center in that it deals with your gut instincts; the things you can stomach and the things you can't. In power this is your healthy ego, out of power it can be swayed and dragged along by others, forever seeking approval or conversely having the need to be in control.

Will Power

As with any energy center the Solar Plexus can be under-active, it may be over-active or it could be in balance. In truth it is probably all of these states at some point during every day.

Once again this chakra draws on the energy from the two either side of it: the heart center and the emotional center. Taken to extremes it can want to bend others to its will; to boss them around to achieve its own objectives. In a position of management, that kind of discipline may be necessary at times but if that same attitude is taken home to children and family it may not be quite so appropriate or nice to be around.

Power

This chakra is like our own version of the sun - it shines. And our entire strength and world comes from the light of the sun. This is an important and vital center. It's about our strength and sustenance; this is our strength of spirit, our resolve and our own ability to shine.

A life time of hard knocks and disappointment can lead to a much diminished energy here. And sometimes you will notice physical indicators of imbalance. Excess weight around the stomach area, (well anywhere actually) can indicate a subconscious need for protection, fat after all is a reserve to call on, in tough times, it's a layer of protection, a comfort. Physical problems with the lower to mid back area, stomach and digestion may also indicate an energy imbalance here.

It's from this chakra you give energy to your wishes and wants, this is the fuel to make things happen, this will spark the ideas. This energy center is given the element of fire. Think about the sun as the fireball, the energy source, the heat source and keep in mind how that can relate to our modern world and the way we live our life today. In this way, your readings will be so much more relevant and accurate for people. This is where our get up and go resides.

Psychic Center

The gut has its own 'brain' and it's this intelligence which is implicated here. This is taking in all that information that your conscious mind on its own can't handle. It can be in knots and very tense at times. It also connects with the kidneys and adrenal glands. If your body is not happy, it will make itself known here.

This is often overlooked as a psychic center, but just as a physical cord attached us to our mother, an ethereal cord attaches us here to our spirit. Feeding this chakra in energetic terms can help to pull in vital reserves to feed our entire energy system.

The Heart Chakra

The Heart Chakra relates to the color green. Obviously here at the heart we are dealing with love, not just of the usual relationship kind though. Almost more importantly is the kind of relationship we have with ourselves. This center can show signs of an eternal giver, a carer or healer, they may be looking after everyone else's needs and not quite so good at looking after their own. This is about giving and sharing but also about **receiving** love.

This center links with the heart as a physical organ but also the level of oxygen in the blood and the lungs themselves, also the circulation of the entire body. I've often picked up whether or not the lungs are affected by smoking here, even if there are no outward signs the person smoked. You may get a sense of congestion and clogginess around this area of the body, if this is the case.

The Throat Chakra

Associated with the color blue, the Throat Chakra is obviously all about the throat and the voice. It includes the neck as well as the mouth and the ears. This is our physical voice but also our spiritual, authentic voice. Do we speak our truth; are we living in line with our authentic personality?

Does the person say what they feel or do they stifle their words, their thoughts and their feelings? This is also the center for change; is change welcomed, or is it resisted and feared? You may get insights and impressions regarding such things when you read the energy in this area.

The neck is the bridge between the mind and the body, a channel of nerves and pathways, very narrow and sensitive. It can be the most vulnerable chakra in a way.

Communication

With this energy center, it is all about communication. Which is not just speaking, although speaking and presenting may be a large part of their life, in as much as they may act or speak for a living in the form of presentations if there is a lot of blue in the aura.

But communication is also about listening and then understanding. There is an inner dialogue going on all the time too; this is about a quiet wisdom. An inner knowing, feeling in tune with your intuition that speaks to you quietly yet constantly. There is a deep and subtle form of communication going on every second.

Third Eye Chakra

The Third Eye is probably the most well known chakra and may be referred to as the psychic center. Located just above and between the eyebrows, it rests in the middle of the forehead. This center resonates with the color indigo.

It links directly to our imagination, which sits hand in hand with our subconscious mind; yet to be fully appreciated or understood. It is thought that our mind has the creative ability to visualize and manifest, if only we would take a minute to believe so.

The Crown Chakra

Located right at the very top of the skull, this is where energy is drawn down into the body from above. This is about our connection to all things. Are we connected or are we isolated? This chakra is associated with Violet and sometimes White.

15 START READING AURAS

To successfully start reading auras, the most helpful piece of advice I can give you is to get out of your own way! Now of course I mean that in the nicest possible sense.

A lot of people and I include myself in this, when they start any psychic related discipline have a myriad of doubts and concerns, wondering whether they are really capable of connecting as they don't think they were born with 'the gift'. Let's clear that up, right now. We all have the ability to tap into and use our intuition, which is our psychic sense. As with anything, without practice or use, you can hardly expect to be an expert in minutes!

Your sixth sense or intuition is in there, you may have different names for it, you may not have noticed it thus far or you may not talk about it very much, but quietly, inside, you know there is more to you than meets the eye. It tends to be a sense we don't use very much and we can then easily doubt or misinterpret its messages and signals.

Reading auras is a perfect way to use your natural psychic ability more and to start engaging some of that unused brain power, we are always reading about. This is about bringing some of that subconscious ability and knowing up into conscious awareness. If you have the desire and interest in the topic, you are already part way there.

So, if you have any doubts at all, just acknowledge them and then put them aside - just for now. One thing you *will* want is an open mind, a clean slate if you like. If you come to topics such as this with massive expectations and preconceived ideas, you will erect your own barriers and hurdles.

Just accept that the doubts are there and decide you'll give it a good go, anyway. If after genuine practice and trial, those concerns win out, then you have lost nothing but what if there *is* more to you, what if you *can* strengthen your connection and intuition? What if reading auras and energy for people, opens doors for you and them - just as it has done for me?

To know that I have reminded people they have a spirit and possibly opened a previously closed or forgotten doorway, always gladdens my heart and makes me feel so privileged. I don't think there is anything more precious you can share with a complete stranger! Our conversations may begin about aura colors and general interest but that then usually leads on to the bigger realization of what the energy can store and hold and that it doesn't start and end with this current life they are experiencing right now.

So, with your clean slate approach, as to your own history and abilities, we can now move on. It was important to share with you some of the many attributes and characteristics of the main aura colors. There are of course more, but those will tend to be mixes of the colors you have already encountered here. Just as in painting, when 2 different colors merge they form a new color, well just consider the individual character traits and how they might merge too.

Don't try and learn the attributes all individually, there is no need. A good way to start is to create a 'typical' Red or Orange Personality type in your mind, as an image - maybe someone you know or have seen on the TV, get to know this personality type as a character and it will be easier for you to recall, rather than have a list of possible facts to remember.

This basic knowledge is going to give you a wonderful grounding, because it will give you a starting point. The hardest thing I found was to just get started and allow my mouth to start speaking. What I found was, when I could push my mind and all its thoughts and imagined worries aside, I could concentrate on the characteristics I knew and was happy with.

Then suddenly a beautiful flow of information and energy started, becoming more of a channel so that the message for the client just naturally came through. Each person was different and will be for you, but I would start with the basic characteristics and as I got into the flow, the information just kept on coming. My mind being free from the hurdles of self doubt, it became a clear path; fresh and relevant images would just come streaming in. All I had to do then was to relate what I saw or felt to the person in front of me.

The sort of things I would see was always different, sometimes I'd get an impression of a relative, particularly if it was relating to a certain issue, and sometimes that impression might be about their own character. Often I would get symbols or images from Tarot cards to household objects. I would have no idea of what might come up before I started; I had just learnt to trust that I would see what was relevant or right for the client.

I would start with the color and as I looked deeper into it and almost conversed with that color, it would change into images and impressions which then changed into mini video clips. My only problem at times, is getting my mouth to keep up, as it can be hard to get the right words for the images I am seeing and sensing as so much information comes in from all directions. It's like all your senses are buzzing and you can only use one of them to tell other people about it.

At first I would wonder if I was making it up (or going mad), but people were confirming the things I said, which gave me confidence to continue. I also realized that I wasn't just seeing an image - I would get a feeling and sensation about it too, which would often unravel more of the story. I knew I wasn't making up how I was feeling and so I just allowed it to flow.

Permission

With the right attitude and mindset, the next thing you want to ensure is that you have the person's permission. This may seem strange but I believe it is not ethically right to go probing unannounced or uninvited into anybody else's energy. You wouldn't do it with anything else they own, so don't do it here.

This is as simple as checking with the person verbally and also checking in non-verbally with your own intuition and/or spirit guides if you are aware of them and work with them already on some level.

If you would like a meditation to find and connect with your own spirit guide, check out the link on the resources page at the end of the book.

Protection

Many people also like to feel protected when doing any kind of energy work. This can open up a whole can of worms and the bigger debate is for other places than here. I personally know I am always protected and feel safe, I know I am a spirit in a body and that my energy is strong and true. But then I have done a lot of energy work, from working with past life energy, negative energy removal and am also a Reiki Master.

The very word protection, suggests you have something to fear, which is probably not the best way to look at it, as often like attracts like in the energy world. Better to think of it as a means to boost your existing energy, so that any unwelcome or unwanted energy does not latch itself onto you, it is merely transmuted into something beautiful and that by raising your energy, you also become a clearer channel, so you have clearer messages and a lot less 'white noise' around. It puts you in a better position, energetically speaking. And you won't feel drained afterwards.

In the beginning, especially if you just want to work with family and friends, you may like to use a simple but effective energy booster or protection visualization. There's a link to free one for you to download and listen to in the resource section of this book.

If you prefer to read instructions, here's a quick guide:

Get yourself in a comfortable seated position, with your feet firmly touching the floor. Take a couple of relaxing breaths, to blow out any tension or unnecessary thoughts and then take your attention within.

Close your eyes and as you breathe in, notice a tiny speck of light, deep in the pit of your stomach. Concentrate on that speck of light and notice how with every breath you take, it expands and grows.

The light can be any color that feels right for you; the most popular tend to be gold, white or silver.

See that light expand until it fills your entire body, from your head to your toes, notice that it feels good, that it almost makes you smile, it feels that good.

Then see that light expand even further, so that it comes past the layer of your skin and forms an aura of sparkling light energy around you. This feels good, strong and very positive. You can make this energy field as large as you like, you may like to add a silver layer to the external edge.

This bright, shining light can only attract more bright, shining light. You feel safe, strong, happy and secure within it. You can hold this for as long as you like, knowing you can recall it at any time.

With practice, this kind of visualization takes minutes, even seconds. You can do it any time you need a boost or even to help you in daily stressful situations. It's great to use if you work in a not so friendly environment - you'll find people bother you a lot less. It's also great to do, to ground, center and balance yourself before you attempt to read anybody's aura. This is one way of clearing your slate, ready to start interpreting the impressions you'll be getting.

Intention

The next thing you will want to consider is setting your intention. Your intention might be to give an entertaining and accurate reading, with both of you enjoying it. Thinking about the outcome you would like, for you and your client, seems to send out a request that often gets answered!

Grounding

With any energy work, we usually have some kind of grounding process, which you can do before or after the reading. This can be a visualization of roots coming out of your feet, going deep into the ground. Some people like to have a drink of water or wash their hands, some will want to physically get up and walk around, maybe rubbing or clapping their hands together.

Reading

At last we can start with the reading!

I like to use the body matrix which I cover in more detail in the next chapter. I usually start with the aura as a whole. I scan the area to see if anything stands out (depending on my intention for the reading).

Then I move from around the feet and work my way up the body. I describe the colors I see and start mentioning the corresponding attributes that come to mind. The rest then just unfolds.

You might sense a color is dull or patchy; this will indicate a lower energy and will correspond with the weaker version of that color's attributes.

You might feel there are holes or energy drains in some areas, using the matrix can help to determine what or who they are. If they are on the right side for example, they could be male, if they are high or behind, then they are often adults. If they are smaller and in front, they are often children. An energy drain is not necessarily a bad thing; it could just be a sign of energy being given out to that person at the moment.

This is one area where you will develop your own style of reading as it depends on whether you sense, see or feel.

Location

It's not just the colors that are important, it's the location and the sense that you get with that, although this is certainly not set in stone, I have found that the matrix is a handy tool to use.

One really strong memory for me and I suspect for the client and her family is one lovely lady who came with her husband on the recommendation of her adult son and his wife, who had both come to see me a few days before.

As usual I started with my initial impressions and described her core color and attributes. There was a lot of blue in her aura, not a full and vibrant shade, in fact in patches it was quite grey and looked worn out. As I got into the flow of things, I had a distinct impression of seeing a leather belt in her aura; it was hovering above her right shoulder.

I didn't have to say very much, as you can probably imagine, I simply relayed what I could see, and as I did, I said, I also felt it was connected to an older male and it felt like that would be her father. Her tears started falling, silently and as I asked her if she wanted to stop, she shook her head and said she wanted to talk about it.

She had just sat and watched me, with her son and his wife, for about an hour working with her husband's aura. She hadn't expected this to come up or even considered it to be possible, but now that it had, she wanted to talk with me about it and she was happy for her family to listen. She had never spoken much about her past and her relationship with her father and how poorly she had been treated.

I think all of us were in tears that afternoon, but there was the most wonderful feeling in the room of being listened to and supported and the four of them stayed for some time. All of us felt humbled and knew that something special had taken place.

So you see, reading auras is not just about entertainment, particularly for me. I want it to be of real help to people, at the same time, I don't expect or look for such deep revelations. It's just a level that I seem to work at and feel happy with. When I gave public demonstrations, I always kept things light and would often just have fun.

What we need to remember is, not everyone with a blue aura will have that same story, all I did was start with the color and as I concentrated on that, more information became visible. It's like reading a book, you have to start by reading the first words on the page, as you keep reading, you work your way through the chapter and the story is slowly revealed.

Reading the aura is the same, except your pages are pages of color, rather than pages of words. This might seem difficult but believe me it's not, what starts as color, soon reveals images, which then reveal that individual's personal story. Don't try and cheat and don't expect a version of War *and Peace* for every person you read for. See it as a bonus. Sometimes the images don't come or are very slow and patchy but if you know that the potential is there for a lot more information, you won't be overwhelmed by it all.

What's important is that you are aware of what can come up and you need to be sensitive to that. Again, you can set this in your intention before you start; that things are kept light hearted yet relevant to the person.

As a rule, I think we only get things come up that we can handle or deal with, for instance, because of my past life training I will often get things that relate to that topic and I love working with the spirit and the soul, so there is always scope for deep and involved work.

If you keep your intentions light at the beginning, should anything come up that requires another professional, whether energy work or counseling etc, you should always refer people and it is good practice to have a list of names you are happy to recommend. This is probably more likely if you want to read auras on a more serious level, again with friends and family, just have fun practicing, to get clearer on what you sense and see.

It can be really interesting and often stimulates people into wanting to find out more about our energetic system and the potential that surrounds and inhabits every human being. Reading auras is not about healing or 'fixing' people, it's about reading auras; reading the energy, which basically is just a way of confirming that our energy body exists.

That is the beauty of it and one of the reasons why I'm interested in the aura. It's a perfect doorway to understanding more about ourselves and ultimately being able to manage our own energy and even healing ourselves; living in balance more of the time.

It may start with just a mild interest and done in the spirit of fun, but when they realize how accurate and true it can be, people are intrigued to find out more for themselves, so a journey begins.

16 THE MAGIC MATRIX

The aura is not something hovering magically outside of us, although that is how we have to draw it. No, it is within and beyond the body; it is made of the fluid energy that connects us all. Encompassing our thoughts, experiences past, present and future potential, they are all there. It holds a million energetic messages and speaks a language we have simply not spoken that much, but just as our eyes see and our ears hear, we as humans have the ability to read and interpret that energy.

You see the physical person in front of you but as you start to work with auras you also see the energetic blueprint and the areas that feel low or high in energy and the things that relate to that.

The aura itself can be easy to read if you use a matrix. After practising and working with this, you may develop your own template but for now I'll share with you mine;

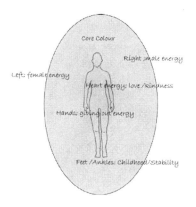

Imagine the aura around the human body, almost as if the body was stood in a very large bubble or goldfish bowl. Actually the goldfish bowl idea works well; the energy we swim in is very similar to water, and you can get a sense of how things blend into each other, there are no fixed and rigid lines.

The color that runs through the middle of the energy system, from top to bottom and around the main body area, is usually your core color. This will be the color that most fits with your personality and you will recognize some of the character traits associated with that. When people talk of aura colors, it is usually this core color that they are referring to.

To read the aura though, it pays to look a little further as particular areas lend themselves to certain types of energy.

Aura Size:

The aura as a whole may feel large and vibrant, it might seem small and withdrawn, and when you initially scan the aura you may or may not get a sense of the overall size and shape.

Left side of the Body:

The left side of the body is feminine energy; this relates to energy coming into your aura, it's what you are taking in. This is important as this is what you absorb, before you then start projecting it out. This is where we can change our energy and aura. If this energy is connected with turmoil and worry, there will usually be something you can do, some steps to take to make things easier or calmer.

Right side of the Body:

The right side is related to male energy. This is more the energy you are giving out - so this is how people will perceive you. There may be a different color to each of the sides.

The Heart:

Around the heart center, you may often pick up a different color or feel to the energy to that of the core. This is all about how we give and receive love. Here is where you might feel that the person is giving out a lot of care and attention and they may need reminding to give themselves some of the kindness they show others.

The Head:

This area is associated with thoughts and beliefs, when reading around the head, you might get a sense of pressure or confusion. If you were to ask the person if they were worried about something at the moment, they would no doubt confirm that they were. The term 'a weight on my shoulders' can literally be sensed in the aura when you start to focus around the head and neck area.

The Hands:

When I focus around the hands, I will often get the sense of energy being given out, streaming away from the person. This area is all about the time and attention we give to things, the things we give our energy to; as that is precisely what we are doing. This is where you then might get a sense of what it is they are pouring their energy into. Often it is connected to children and family.

The Feet:

The energy around the feet is all to do with how we stand, how we perform, how strong we are. If there is an imbalance to the energy here, there is usually something going on in their life that is causing them to feel unstable. This can be a move of home or job for example. By the feet I may also get a sense of childhood issues and events.

Behind:

The energy behind the person you are reading for, often relates to the past or people older than the client: I usually pick up parents here - particularly if the energy is *still* being affected by their parents. To be more precise, they are stood behind but to the side and usually the father or male energy stands to the right and the mother and female energy stands to the left.

Often if their partner is domineering or if a parent has been controlling then I may get a sense of that causing the energy of the person I am reading for to bend away or over to the side.

In Front:

The area in front of you, relates to your future. Predictions are not really my thing but we can change our future as we change our thoughts and beliefs. You may get a sense of gifts being given here or a celebration that might be happening soon. When you start to focus on this future energy, you will usually scan in front and above the person and then get a sense of what is to come.

I've put the body matrix and the core characteristics into a PDF you can print off and download, so you don't have to worry about remembering everything. There's a link to it on the resource page.

17 SEEING, SCANNING & SENSING AURAS

Although our main concern with this book is how to read an aura, and there is lots of information available about seeing one, I thought I'd share with you a bit more about how I go about it.

If you have an aura image taken already, you can work with that and now hopefully understand the colors in it a little more. Or, you might like to see what you can pick up from a photo.

Alternatively, if you have a real, live person to read for, here are a few tips that might help you tune into your senses a little bit more:

Seeing

As I said before, don't expect to see it with your eyes, certainly not immediately. What you can do though, is get a sense of it, an impression: in effect seeing it with your mind's eye. This isn't just idle imagination, you will know on a gut level if it feels right, or you might get other images and sensations that will lead you to something of relevance to the person in front of you.

Scanning

First I do an overall scan. Having set my intention, I look at the area around the body, to see what I feel. I'm not expecting images, it's like I'm just looking at and feeling the energy, even if I am stood yards away. I'm feeling for the vibrancy and the flow. For example I might get an impression of it being pulled and twisted to one side, maybe even being held back.

If something stands out or pulls your attention you work with that. How do you work with it? You ask questions! All done in your mind, although you can speak them out loud if that feels right for you. It sounds a little crazy, but try it; you'll find that is when the answers and other images come. This is similar to how a medium works; you might hear them say, "Ok, show me more" or "What does that relate to?" We can do the same things here.

If you don't ask questions and have a dialogue, you can't have a conversation - it's as simple as that. Remember, this is your energy, your subconscious mind reaching out and touching theirs. It's all done with your thought and intention, that's how you send the ripple of a message out. When it returns it usually has some feeling, sentiment or emotion in it - it now has a different flavor and essence: that of the other person.

After I've got an overall sense, I will then check on the core area, as people love to know what color they are. I often start from the feet up and check that core channel, to determine the color and again if there are any energy shifts or things that stand out there.

I might ask more questions;

- How are the feet, the shoes, the legs, what does the energy feel like?
- If the toes could talk what would they be saying?
- Are they squashed, are they pinched, do they look happy and at ease, are they looked after?

Don't discount anything, everything talks to you.

I once read a pair of shoes for a lady. She had no idea that's what spoke to me, but when I had initially scanned her energy field, they really stood out and my attention kept being pulled to them. They were the kind with lace up ribbons around the ankle. I focused on the shoes and it's a bit like then blurring your vision (sometimes I might even close my eyes as our external vision can often distract us) but I wasn't looking at them thinking about their color or fit so much as what story did they have to tell me? I asked "Why are you here?"

The next thing was I got a sense of ballet, and an image of the woman as a child dancing and loving it. There was an innocence to the feeling and a sense of lightness and fun. Everything was very pink and reminded me of the Barbie doll. This was very different to how the lady was now sat, her demeanor and expression.

I sensed this was how she had been as a child, this is what her spirit longed for again, but something had caused her life to be different. To me she now felt restricted and tied; that sense of freedom was bursting to get out and yet it just couldn't.

I relayed this to her and her husband, who was sitting next to her. He answered for her, as she was a little upset. Apparently this was the first time in a long while that she had ventured outside. She rarely left the house these days. She had really wanted to come to our meeting though and had made a mammoth effort to get there.

She herself then started to speak, yes she had danced as a child and yes she had loved it. Apparently she had loved Barbie as a young girl and her bedroom had been like a Barbie palace and shrine. Several incidents had happened in her life since then, that now made her feel scared to leave the house. She went on to explain more and at the end of the evening she felt like a weight had been lifted. Although she understood there was more to do, she felt positive for the first time that things could change for the better.

To me, it wasn't about anything mystical and having her aura read; it was more to do with her own spirit yearning for life, for change. She resonated with the people there, strangers who showed her kindness, understanding and compassion, without judgment or blame. It was a safe space for her to explore.

I was hardly likely to assume that a woman in a group meeting was scared of going outside and wouldn't normally leave the house. If it's in your energy you can't hide it, one thing with energy I forgot to mention, it doesn't lie. We can interpret it wrongly, but it will never lie.

That to me is the beauty of reading auras; it's not the entertainment factor, although that on its own can be great fun. It opens a doorway to the spirit, whether people realize it or not. That's who I talk to, that's who speaks to me, and then I as the person, deliver that message back to the individual in terms they can relate to.

Sensing

It will depend on you which of your senses you might use or be strongest in. There is no right or wrong one. Sometimes if I was combining a Reiki session with the reading, I would be much closer and physically use my hands to scan the energy field.

Then I would get definite feelings in my hands, for example one chap's energy was all fine and I wasn't feeling anything much to start with. As he was laying down I had started from his head. Then as I moved my hands down to his knees, they felt very cold and it was like there was little or no energy there. My hands were a few inches from his body; I was literally just running my hands through his energy field.

It turned out that he had been a soldier a few years previous and had had serious surgery on his lower legs after a terrible accident.

This kind of energy work is probably easier if you have had some training but your hands are great antennae for picking up energy. You might feel temperature changes; you might get the sensation of pins and needles. It might even feel clammy and sticky. This is where you then will either get a sense of what that means, or if you just mention that you felt an energy change in the area, the person will often know what the cause is.

The things that are irrelevant won't draw you in, the aspects with a story to tell, will, they are itching to let you know. I think that what blocks a lot of people is they expect to get messages or impressions in a certain way.

Just allow the images and sensations to come in, exactly as you do with beautiful music you listen to, your ears may be listening but images and sensations are conjured up in your mind. So it is with reading auras, be as unattached as you would be listening to music, you simply flick the switch that says you are ready to listen. Don't force the sound, just let it come and allow your mind to fill. Instead of sound we are working with energy and color, feelings and vibrations, it's like appreciating a beautiful work of art. Each of us is a unique canvas and just as you can read a painting, you can read the aura.

Unless you're a healer, read - don't heal. Inevitably my readings often resulted in some form of healing as that is what I am trained to do. Don't try and fix people, ideally it's about everyone being able to discover more about their aura and energy system, then finding out what ways work for them to find balance. Just as we as adults can decide what food we eat and monitor our diet and physical health, so we can monitor our energetic heath too.

Reading auras is not about you having power over others, it is an absolute privilege and should always be treated as such.

Sensitivity

What I've found, is that people are surprised to know, just what can be seen and felt in the aura by a complete stranger. Because I handle the situation sensitively they are often prompted then to take action to help them deal with whatever has come up;

Two ladies came to the center where I was working one day, to meet for coffee and thought it might be a bit of fun to have their aura read! One of the ladies had no energy from the ankles down, it was as if it had been chopped off, it felt like a very sharp line, which is unusual.

I told her what I felt and that I thought it related to her childhood and that it was her that had pushed it away, she was the one who had drawn that line. That was it, the tears were falling. It turned out that this was completely true and she had not wanted to talk to anyone about it before but recently she had been thinking that she would like to find someone to work with, to help her understand it and work through it.

After a very shocked coffee break, she came back to me and said she wasn't quite ready to do anything straight away but she felt she had found the person who she could feel safe enough with to help her and that it was me. Obviously I was very touched and agreed to help as much as I could and refer her to other professionals if and when the time should come.

At that time I was working from a courtyard setting with several shops and a tea room. The lady from the shop next door asked me one day what exactly it is I did to people. I asked what she meant and she said.

"Well, they come to you, they walk in all normal, but when they leave they look like they've been crying, then they all hug you and seem to love you for it!" We both laughed at that - I hadn't thought about how it must look from the outside but she was so right in how she had described it.

This is not my intention, I do not seek to make people cry nor impress them with great revelations. The tears just tend to happen, more often than not as I trust that what is right and relevant for them, is what will make itself known to me. I will only broadly touch on topics or areas in a reading as any deeper issues and concerns are best dealt with by a qualified person in an appropriate setting.

Often people wanted to take up therapy with me, as they felt safe to trust, confide and open up - especially as we had already started talking about the issue in a non confrontational or therapeutic way. If it was not in my area of expertise I would always refer people to appropriate professionals.

This may not happen to you, it pays to be aware though of the sensitive nature of the energy you are working with, this is not entertainment, this is real people's lives, their feelings and their experiences and they should always be treated with respect.

This is how I read auras and if you work with it, then I believe that you too will be reading them soon and that then you may well develop your own energetic dialect that will work just as well for you.

I wish you all the best and hope you allow more color and energy into your life.

In this second edition on the following pages I've added in preview chapters of 2 other titles;

    Chakra Balancing - A Practical Guide to Balancing The Chakras & Start Chakra Healing Today

    &

    Past Lives; Incredible Past Life Experiences

DAVINA

Davina DeSilver

Davina DeSilver

PREVIEW CHAPTERS:

CHAKRA BALANCING - A PRACTICAL GUIDE TO BALANCE THE CHAKRAS & START CHAKRA HEALING TODAY

1 CAN YOU TALK THE LANGUAGE OF ENERGY?

An Introduction to the Chakras:

Chakra is an ancient Sanskrit term, it's translated meaning is 'spinning disc' or 'wheel'. More often than not, when we are talking about the chakras of the human body, we tend to be referring to the main seven chakras of the human energy system. (There are more, but for simplicity we will focus on the main seven here).

Despite the ancient unveiling and naming of the chakras, it has been a relatively recent discovery that each of the major chakras resides very close to an important nerve plexus or center, within the body.

It's important to keep in mind that the chakras are not things you can see or touch, they are not part of your physical body but they *are* part of your energetic body. To me, they are doorways, connecting your conscious and subconscious minds, as well as connecting your energetic and physical body.

The healers and seers of ancient times perceived that these seven major energy hubs or centers, were positioned along the human spine, from the very bottom vertebra, right to the topmost point of the head. They described the energy at these points as spinning. Similar to the motion you see where two volumes of water converge and a whirlpool is created.

The locations of the seven main Chakras are:

- The Base or Root Chakra - The base of the spine
- The Sacral or Second Chakra - The lower abdomen, about a hand width from your navel
- The Third Chakra or Solar Plexus - Resides around the navel and slightly above it
- The Fourth or Heart Chakra - Obviously this is located in the chest area
- The Fifth or Throat Chakra - This energy centre is situated at the throat, and affects the neck region as a whole
- The Sixth Chakra or Third Eye - Located between and slightly above the eyebrows
- The Seventh or Crown Chakra - This uppermost Chakra is positioned at the top of the head

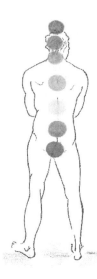

They may not be tangible nor something you have spent a lot of time thinking about but you can certainly become more aware of the existence of the chakra energies. You can become more sensitive to how they feel and then go on to interpret the energetic signals they are constantly giving out.

Every one of the seven chakras vibrates at a unique frequency; its own particular resonance. One of the ways we distinguish them most easily is by color.

- Red is the color of the Root Chakra
- Orange for the Sacral Chakra
- Yellow for the Third Chakra/Solar Plexus
- Green for the Heart Chakra
- Blue for the Throat Chakra
- Indigo for the Sixth Chakra/Third Eye
- Violet for the Seventh/Crown Chakra

The energy of the human body is constantly communicating and therefore has a language. It is a language we can all converse in subconsciously. When you can *consciously* understand and communicate with it, then you are in a position to know yourself at a much deeper level, using and directing energy to sustain and improve your general health and wellbeing.

The energy flows from the main centers along minuscule channels, each nourishing and feeding particular areas of the body. Each center is also associated with the endocrine glands; these regulate many of the main functioning systems of your body, working directly with the hormones. The types of functions affected are: your general energy levels, respiration, reproduction, overall growth and development.

You may have heard about the chakras being out of alignment or balance, maybe even closed. They are constantly regulating your energy, attempting a state of homeostasis, just as the physical body does. Your energetic 'body' is doing the same; it wants a balanced and stable sense of equilibrium. It will strive to maintain a sense of balance as best it can. Being in balance is the optimum healthy state.

The chakras can reveal themselves as being out of balance in a variety of ways. They may spin very slowly, almost unevenly, they may run very fast. The energy can feel weak or may be backing up, coming to a head. A bit like most things in life, we can get away with it for a while. Having an out of balance chakra may not appear to be too significant or important. But as in life, everything does have an effect and compensations will be made, energy may be taken from other sources, and other areas may start to be affected.

Our energy system is similar to our immune system, it can be strong or weak, and any point in between! It is constantly working for our optimum performance and protection. It is possible and in my opinion, more than likely, that a weaker chakra center is where a physical symptom or problem is going to find it easiest to take hold. It may be in the form of an illness or disease or stress and tension or even an accident and injury.

Metaphysically speaking, areas of the body reveal psychosomatic symptoms and triggers, which can reveal the underlying implications of what is really going on. This is intricately connected with your subconscious thoughts, what your subconscious <u>believes</u> to be true and the subsequent messages it is giving your body. When our minds take hold of something as true, regardless of whether it actually **is** a truth or not, it sets a chain of actions in motion, to reinforce that thought and make it a concrete reality.

It's not just your mind that the chakras connect to. They are also in constant communication with your mental health and emotional wellbeing, not to mention the spiritual aspect of your being. They can reveal so much about us, on so many levels. Regular attention to the chakras and your energy system as a whole can help you achieve a much better level of overall health and a sense of holistic wellbeing.

One thing is a given. Your energy speaks the truth - it doesn't lie. It doesn't smooth over the cracks or say what it thinks you might want to hear - it is quietly broadcasting 24 hours a day in subtle ways - and what it communicates is always the truth.

This is one of the reasons I love energy work so much - it's a bit like working with animals, it is what it is and it does what it does. It is very pure and simple, if there is an imbalance or weakness, it will show it. The magic is in deciphering what it is revealing and that requires an honest and open mind.

In this book, we cover a general, broad overview of the main energy centers and indicators of what it would feel like to be in balance for each chakra. We also highlight some of the most common signs and symptoms of imbalance. Then you'll find there are a few suggestions of simple and practical ways to bring balance back to each one of your chakras.

By the time you've finished, you will be well on your way to learning to speak the language of energy. I've deliberately kept it short, to the point and easy to read, so you can get started right away.

2 IT'S NOT JUST ABOUT BALANCE

Tip the Energy Scales in Your Favor

Don't waste your time on a one - off balance. It's simply not enough.

Lots of people think they are helping themselves by getting into the chakras and think that the odd chakra balance or energy treatment is going to do the job. Just as one trip to the hairdresser won't keep your style looking good for long, neither will the odd half-hearted energy balance. But don't be put off either. There are a great many simple yet effective things you can do and probably to a degree already are doing that can really help your energy system.

The more you make things simple and easy, the more likely you will be able to sustain them and reap the long term benefits. If you can also make your energy work enjoyable, then you'll probably find the time to fit it into your busy schedule. So then it becomes a part of your regular routine.

The chakras are an integral part of your health. To remain physically healthy you need to eat and act healthily - it is exactly the same with your energetic health. For optimum effect incorporate chakra balancing, breath work or meditating as a part of your regular daily or weekly routine. It shouldn't be a chore as it can be an extremely enjoyable and relaxing, totally therapeutic process! You certainly don't want to be too compulsive or regimental about it either, energy work needs to flow and be fluid. It should be a natural and enjoyable part of your week, that's why I like to include practical and simple methods as they are far more likely to get done.

Not many of us live our lives in balance all the time, floating on a lovely fluffy cloud just above 'real world land'. No, we live in the modern world, with all the wonderful things it brings as well as all the not so wonderful. We have demands on our time, our energy, our pockets and our patience. Keep things as real and practical and as easy to do as you can. To start with, try swapping 30 minutes of TV time for a meditation or relaxation class. The benefits to your body can be immediate.

In a deep state of relaxation, the mind can be so receptive and immensely powerful. It is a direct route to tap into our amazing potential of healing and creativity. Successful business people, sports men and women the world over, use the power of their mind to achieve all sorts of amazing things in their lives. A great many people have healed themselves of all manner of different illnesses and diseases. You don't need to wait until you're unwell to harness this power.

We all have the ability and the potential. For many of us though, it can seem counter intuitive to take time out from our busy lives and if we don't see an immediate effect we decide it's not working and go back to old habits and routines. We get comfortable in our discomfort. It doesn't have to be that way.

Harness the power of your core, your inner self and your chakra energy to find the clarity of thought, the peace of mind and the wisdom to live your life more fulfilled, happy and at ease than you ever imagined was possible. Just make it more likely to happen by establishing new, fun habits that feed and nourish you. Things that balance your energy and positively feed it, without you having to think too much about it.

Learn to speak the language of energy and understand what it is trying to tell you.

Chakra Energy - Where Does it Come From?

There is energy all around us, in everything we can see and in everything we can't. There's energy in the trees, in plants, in our lights and buildings. There's energy in nature herself, trees have a different energy to mountains, and the sea has a different energy to earth. Many people are familiar with crystals and can appreciate that they each have their own unique energy too. Everything has its own special frequency, even every individual plant and flower. It is this energy that makes homeopathy and aromatherapy so successful. So already you can see we are swimming in a universal soup of energy, we can't not be affected by it. This is how we are all connected. Not joined at the hip but swimming in the same big pond.

It doesn't stop there; each and every organ in the body and every illness have a different energy too. It's not just your physical movements and actions that have a frequency and an energetic effect, your words and thoughts do too.

Everything has its own unique frequency and energy vibration

This might seem a little hard to take but consider how you feel when you hear a beautiful hymn or a Christmas carol being sung. It lifts your spirit and makes you feel good inside. Now how does it feel when you hear harsh words? It usually sparks a completely different reaction inside. It doesn't feel good at all and it might even spark a fearful reaction in you. There is energy in those words, in their feeling and emotion. Emotions are our most powerful energy transmitters. We are reacting on an energetic level all the time. The chakras are our energy hubs; they constantly take in this energy and release it out.

As you might expect, some things are good for your energy and some things are not so great. Some things feed you and some detract from you. You will already have a pretty good idea of what does and doesn't work for you, even if you haven't outwardly acknowledged it before. You may even have noticed that some places feel comfortable and ok with you and some seem to make you feel on edge or your skin crawl. What is attractive and appealing to one, will not necessarily be the same for the next person. It is precisely because the energies are continually fluctuating, in and out that we need to understand them better. If we can work in harmony for more of the time and less against the flow, the better off we all will be.

If you can imagine the exchange of energy is as vital and as integral as breathing - in and out, in and out, 24- 7,then you can appreciate that a one - off energy balance won't do much good. Find ways that you know work for you, try some of the things I mention in this book, some you'll like and be drawn to and some you won't. What matters is you find what works for you, and the things you know feed your energy, without having to drastically alter your life or abstain from the modern world and all it has to offer.

Davina DeSilver

PAST LIVES:

INCREDIBLE PAST LIFE EXPERIENCES

1 INTRODUCTION

I have been shocked, elated, stunned and at times frozen with fear.

These are my experiences, never anyone famous, just real experiences of past lives, usually, though not always, with some pertinent reminder or similarity with events in my current life.

Can I prove the existence of past lives, no am I going to try, no - this is just a simple sharing about the things I have, seen and felt. I am no actress and no prima donna, in fact I hate fuss and bother of any kind, had I known I was going to be reeling about convinced I was in pain or crying so much in front of a crowd of fellow students I probably would never have signed up for the course. But a part of me wanted to know. I wanted to know for real, not be told about it by someone else.

Believing in the philosophy of 'better out than in' and being a bit of a natural skeptic I also knew I would only truly believe if I experienced things for myself. If things came up that needed to be dealt with, I didn't want to pretend they weren't there or sweep them under the carpet, I was ready to let go.

2 PAST LIFE REGRESSION THERAPY

My experiences of the existence of past lives have never been for entertainment purposes. I have loved being able to touch my spirit and that of others. Within all of us, lies the potential to access ancient memories, and times long past. I do believe that the body holds onto such memories, even if we don't consciously know how.

There is an intelligence in every single cell of our bodies. The mind is not the brain, it includes the brain but it is not limited to it. The brain is the physical organ, the mind is less tangible. It expands further than we think and communicates in ways I believe we have yet to master or fully understand.

There may be things in this life that just don't make sense to you, a recurring thought or dream that seems to bear no relevance to your current life. Sometimes specific aches, pains and physical imbalances may not be confined to an event in this current lifetime. If that is the case for you, you will know it in your heart *and* in your gut as you read these words. Using the sensations and feeling ability of the body is one of the ways we can access these deeply held memories, thoughts and beliefs. It's as if they are frozen in time, crystallized if you like, especially if they are associated with strong emotions and events.

The emotions, thoughts and beliefs at the time of death are particularly important and telling. Just as the consciousness of a baby responds to life and sounds outside of the womb before birth so does our consciousness at the point of death... and beyond.

As the soul experiences lifetime after lifetime, these strong residual memories can also be recreated; a chronic throat condition may relate to a previous hanging or strangulation. A frozen shoulder might correspond with an old bullet wound for example or an irrational fear of water might suggest a previous experience of drowning. These things may not make much sense in your modern day context but the energy behind them can be holding you back from living a peaceful life.

Such memories can be brought into our conscious awareness by different emotional states; by depression or anxiety, stress and phobias, even recurring relationship difficulties, nightmares and obsessions. I certainly found this to be true not only for myself but in others too. It's as if an energetic ripple from the past slowly edges in, to make itself known in some way in our current life. When we recognize it for what it is and are drawn to regression, we can follow the tell tale threads that reverberate in this life and find ourselves in times long since past; tasting an experience we thought was long forgotten.

I know in my heart what I have experienced in my own past life experiences and that of my fellow students and clients is true. I have never entered a past life seeking proof; I suppose I have been much more selfish than that. I wanted to feel it for myself, I wanted understanding and I wanted to feel the truth of it. I didn't want to enter the process with preconceived ideas or specific expectations.

I was prepared to walk away knowing I had tried it, if it turned out to be false or a little too flaky for me. At the time of my life I took my training, I believe the work I did with my spirit and soul ultimately helped me to become much more rounded and not only more nurturing and protective of my own energy but that of others too.

3 IT'S NOT FOR EVERYONE

Regression is not for everyone and it is not a magical elixir to solve every problem we have. But it can be very profound and will certainly suit some more than others. If it appeals to you, I am sure the opportunity will arise for you to experience it. When there is a pulling in your heart and the thought just won't seem to go away that is usually a good indicator it will be of use to you.

For me, regression therapy started a wonderful journey of working with spirit. I qualified with my diploma in regression therapy first and only then did I start my hypnosis training. I studied energy and became a Reiki Master and that lead on to all sorts of other energy related workshops and seminars, from reading auras to dealing with negative entities. Even to working with the tarot, not so much as a means of divination but I love how the images reveal profound insights about our consciousness and the story of life and how we evolve and grow over time.

In this book, I share a few of my experiences and on occasion use quotes taken directly from class notes recorded by my fellow pupils at the time. It's a combination of sharing the past life, whilst explaining a little about the technique and psychology behind it so you can see how the experience can be of benefit to those that find the idea appealing.

Contra Indicators

There are some instances where regression is not recommended and should even be avoided; the most common are listed below. It is always worth checking these out before considering past life regression.

People unable to think rationally and clearly, severely depressed, anorexic or schizophrenic symptoms, people taking high dosages of anti depressants or anti anxiety drugs.

Heart problems or fits and seizures can also be prohibitive as some memories can hold a lot of charge, invoking powerful emotions and sensations.

4 WHAT IS PAST LIFE REGRESSION THERAPY?

How do we remember and where do we store those memories? These are such big questions that could keep the greatest minds debating for lifetimes. There is no definitive short answer, things that we think are long forgotten can be recalled by any of our senses; sound, smell, taste, touch or sight.

They can be stored in the depths of our minds for years, seemingly dormant until a catalyst reawakens them. Many of our experiences and memories hold no specific charge for us and can be pleasant warm recollections, some however can not only hold an emotional charge but they can also be destructive or limiting in some way.

Often it is not the memories themselves but the associations and connections we add to them that make them restrictive or limiting. To an outsider these can seem irrational, even ridiculous yet they are all so real to the person involved.

It is when such thoughts are unhelpful to our current lives that regression can be helpful.

Past life regression is a technique used to gain access to these deepest memories and resonances, whether real or imagined.

Once they are accessed and the underlying story revealed, a new level of understanding can be attained. Not only understanding, for when we use regression as a therapy we go beyond merely watching the scene. We work with it, employing specific techniques to allow the client to 'put right' or make adjustments to these memories so that they can bring peace and healing to the situation.

In this way, directly communicating with the subconscious mind, there is usually a positive effect noticed in the person's current life. It's as if they have been able to shift a burden in their energy and move on feeling much freer and lighter.

What can it do for me?

Past life regression often works where conventional methods do not or where the symptoms noted do not make much sense. These can be anything from recurring thoughts, problems, dreams or fears. The sort of thing that you know rationally doesn't seem to stack up and yet somehow they just won't go away.

Many therapies use the creative ability of the mind, to provide answers and the stimulus for change. It is here our flashes of insight and inspiration arrive and left unchecked, it is also here that our thoughts can run riot and we can find ourselves worrying about things that in actuality will never happen, yet we allow these fears to block our lives and prevent us from doing so much in life.

NLP uses the positive use of imagery to effect changes in a variety of creative ways; from reducing negative images in our mind to adding color and feeling to the positive images we *do* want. The power of metaphors and the imagery associated with them is also well documented and practiced.

When we communicate with the subconscious mind it does not require facts and figures to make sense of things, its language is much more sensory and visual. Repeated messages are soon embedded and can become beliefs over time. Beliefs are powerful thoughts which underpin much of our lives, some we are consciously aware of and many we are not. The most powerful of these can be the beliefs about ourselves and our ability, our appearance and performance.

The mind holds the key to the store house of these thoughts, memories and beliefs, with new perspectives and understanding we can change many things, we can evaluate and discern. We can make decisions and choices to stay the same or change. In order to do this though, we need to be consciously aware of such thoughts and past life regression can surface them and the associated beliefs, shedding light on long forgotten threads that may well be affecting you today.

Those threads can be untied and rewoven bringing a sense of resolution, completion and peace, not just to a specific situation but to the attitude the subconscious has around it too. This is where you can notice beneficial changes to your everyday life you are experiencing right now.

In a therapeutic setting we accumulate facts and facets of the story which directly relate to the specific symptoms of the client. These are for personal discovery and empowerment and it is important to understand the story of the past life, to be able to navigate it to the point of death in that lifetime and then beyond. For it is in the afterlife that we can spend a great deal of time in the regression session as it is here that we can invite healing and compassionate understanding. This is the aspect I feel, that brings immense peace to clients and it is a wonderful privilege to share that space with them.

As therapists we are not interested in proving what is uncovered by the client, we respect the validity of their experiences, whether real or imagined. Regression sessions can be very powerful, emotive, humbling *and* empowering. It requires a deep level of trust and sharing. To be invited into the inner world that holds so much meaning and importance for the individual is an honor. We work with the imagery of the client's mind however it wishes to present itself, always keeping the goal of the therapy in mind.

There are however many studies that have followed regressions and **have** been conducted with a more fact finding and scientific approach. These studies have traced the facts given by the people regressed to check the validity of statements or claims made where possible. One of the most notable studies being *Twenty Cases Suggestive of Reincarnation* by Dr Ian Stevenson and the story of Arthur Flowerdew whose past life memories helped archaeologists with missing parts of their knowledge of Petra, a city in Jordan.

What can it be used for?

Although we don't need a reason or a symptom to experience a past life, some of the things that have responded well to using regression as a therapy are:

- Depression
- Irrational fears/thoughts
- Phobias & panic attacks
- Re-occurring Relationship Problems
- Experiencing feelings of detachment and separateness
- Flash backs from dreams/ recurring images

"In summary Regression Therapy works with the psychological, somatic and spiritual unresolved residues from our present life and past lives. It is a comprehensive method for transforming them in a way that is both safe and structured." Andy Tomlinson *an Insight into Past Life Regression.*

Resources

Meet Your Spirit Guide Meditation

Empowering & Boosting Your Energy Visualization

The Body Matrix & Key Points PDF

Available at:

http://aurasandchakras.com/resources2

Other Titles By Davina DeSilver

Chakra Balancing - A Practical Guide to Balancing The Chakras & Start Chakra Healing Today

Chakra Awakening - A Beginners Guide to the Chakras

A great introduction and insight into the main seven chakras, how they relate to your life and how to start working with their energy.